The Third Marathon

The objective is to live longer not to kill yourself

Paul Brannigan

Best Wishes

Paul

Copyright © 2024 Paul Brannigan

The right of Paul Brannigan to be identified as the author of this book has been asserted in accordance with the Copyright, Designs and Patents Act 1988

Printed November 2024

First published 2024 by

> Secrets of Success Ltd
> Unit 115
> 155 Minories
> London
> EC3N 1AD
> United Kingdom

All Rights Reserved. No part of this publication may be reproduced, stored in a retrieval system or transmitted in any form or by any means, electronic, mechanical, photocopying, recording, scanning or otherwise, except under the terms of the Copyright, Designs and Patents Act 1988 or under the terms of a licence granted by the Copyright Licensing Agency Ltd, 90 Tottenham Court Road, London, W1T 4LP, without the permission in writing of the publisher.

Designations used by companies to distinguish their products are often claimed as trademarks. The owl logo is the trademark property of the author Paul Brannigan. All other brand names and product names used in this book are trade names, service marks, trademarks or registered trademarks of their respective owners.

This publication is designed to put forward ideas to promote improved health and fitness. The ideas and exercises set out in this book have been tried and tested, and are put forward in good faith. Neither the publishers nor the author can accept responsibility for the loss occasioned to any person acting or refraining from action as a result of the material contained in this book. If professional advice or other expert assistance is required, the services of a competent professional should be sought.

Cover photo: Paul on 2 May 2018, running along *Route de L'Europe* between *Prévessin-Moëns* and *Aire de fitness Bois de Serves*, just north of CERN, Geneva.

Route de L'Europe was affectionately known as "The Fridge".

Whilst it looks glorious in summer, it's freezing cold in winter. The trees along the footpath trap the cold air. No matter the season, you are guaranteed to transition from warmer air to colder air as you enter The Fridge!

Dedication

To

Dr Georges Canguilhem

Prof Richard Trembath

Dr Giles Yeo

Thank you

Contents

Preface ix

Chapters

1	What Exactly Are You Trying to do?	1
2	Everything You Need to Get Started	9
3	Shoes, Shoes and More Shoes	21
4	Training Begins	33
5	Techniques, Stretches and Exercises	41
6	Race Preparation	55
7	Marathon 1 Milton Keynes	65
8	A Modified Training Program	79
9	Marathon 2 Geneva	89
10	Third Time Lucky and Unlucky	105
11	Weight Management and Calories	125
12	Books, Books and More Books	137
13	The Secret Sauce	149
14	Plan Your Marathon	163
15	Marathon 3 Chelmsford	169
16	The Future	181
17	A Letter to My Younger Self	189

Appendices

1	My Why What How	193
2	Example Log	195
3	Example Wiki	197
4	The Golden Rules	199
5	Example Diary - Milton Keynes	203
6	Example Diary - Geneva	205
7	Example Diary - Chelmsford	207
8	Example Pace Sheets	209
9	Race Day Checklist	211
	Bibliography	213
	Index	221

Preface

It takes stamina, physical strength, mental strength and bucketfuls of willpower. Running a marathon is a challenge!

I started incrementally, and did my first 10k race in 2006 when I was 44 years old. Overweight, unhealthy, and determined to do something about it. Then in 2007 I completed my first half marathon. And then I thought, you know what, setting yourself a goal, like a marathon, is a handy way to keep yourself focussed on improving your health and fitness. Isn't it? Setting a goal helps you improve. Hitting the target, helps you set a new goal, which then helps you improve more. A positive self reinforcing feedback loop.

If only there was a book to help me?

This is the book that I first wanted to read in early 2010 when I started serious preparations to run an actual marathon! This is also the book that I wanted to read fourteen years later, in 2024, just before I completed my third marathon.

I've bought "how to" books. I've read many online resources. I've discussed running with staff at the gym, and with people at two different running clubs. All of it has been superficially helpful, though none of it has been particularly detailed. Short of hiring a running coach (which I couldn't afford) I didn't really have the input I needed to plan well, to train well, and to build the persistency and consistency that marathon runners need.

As an amateur runner, it had taken me until 2024 to gather all the right material, to gain enough knowledge to be genuinely instructive, and to write and publish this book. It's partly autobiographical, and partly instructional. It's one man's story of a twenty year journey from fat forty something to fit sixty something.

None of the "how to" books helped me much. They all seemed to assume that I was a twenty something or a thirty something, and that I wanted to achieve a marathon time of something like four hours. I was 40+ and I wanted to finish in less than six hours, just ahead of the sweeper bus.

Amongst all of my stories and anecdotes, this book provides a wide ranging mix of information; comprehensive discussions covering planning, logging and training, details of clothing, shoes, nutrition and diet, and how to handle injuries and weight management. And in spite of the limitations of conveying all of this with no more than text, illustrations and tables, I have tried to weave it all together using generous measures of sincerity and emotional support. If I can do a marathon (or three) then you can probably do a marathon too!

My first 10k and my first half marathon were both small local events. I didn't enjoy the half marathon, and I didn't do well. However, I did finish before the sweeper bus. As I crossed the finish line the thought in my head was "my distance is 10k and I should just stick to doing that".

However, the idea of "doing a marathon" just wouldn't go away, and repeatedly came back to torment me. Well, I'd only have to do just one wouldn't I? And that would put the incessant nagging to bed once and for all wouldn't it?

A marathon is a feat which few people achieve. I cannot tell you where the statistic comes from, nor how authentic it is. Back in 2005 the staff at my gym would often say that only *one half of one percent* of the UK population has ever completed a marathon. Could I join that half a percent?

I also thought that it would be really meaningful to complete my first marathon when I hit a significant personal milestone. As you will learn from Chapter 7, in May 2013 (then aged 50) I did that, the Milton Keynes Marathon. This book tells you how it went, what happened next, and how that led to my second and my third marathons. Chapter 9 discusses the marathon in Geneva in May 2018 (aged 55), and Chapter 15 details the third marathon around Chelmsford in October 2024 (aged 61). The story also explains why I failed to follow the obvious 5 year pattern and decided to not enter a marathon in 2023 when I was 60 years old.

Now what I would like to know is, what percentage of the UK population has completed *two* marathons? Or *three*? And what *you* want to know is, how things progressed in the build up to each of the three marathons? The successive chapters explain all of that in chronological fashion. As you will read in Chapter 16 my future running program remains an open question. It hasn't yet finished.

This book is strictly amateur, written by an amateur runner for amateur runners. With thousands upon thousands of kilometres behind me, I can probably describe myself as a dedicated amateur, though I still feel like I'm a complete novice. There is probably a boundary between novice and amateur, and I seem to be a perpetual resident of that boundary.

They say that you spend your first two marathons learning how *not* to run a marathon. The first twelve chapters of this book were completed before I did the Chelmsford Marathon in October 2024. The closing chapters were written soon after. What you are getting is the full, authentic story of the first two marathons which teach us *how not to run a marathon*, and the third one which may or may not have been much better than the first two. By following this twenty year time line you will learn how the entire history unfolded, and how (even now) I still seem to be hovering in that boundary between novice and amateur.

Hence, you can think of this book as a book which has been written by a novice marathoner for novice marathoners. It's not a recipe for running a marathon. It's a personal story of my disjointed efforts to be a more accomplished marathon runner. Had I wanted to write a concise recipe for you I would have omitted a lot of the anecdotes, shortened the time lines, and deprived you of some of the fun, the fascination and the frustration that I went through.

In a variety of places I have included some personal facts and figures. I apologise if it sometimes comes over as virtue signalling, that was not the intention. The figures are my authentic figures, the brutal facts, and I hope they provide you with some indication of what can genuinely be achieved. They demonstrate what a fat bloke was actually capable of!

This book is for every aspiring marathon runner. However, as an overweight middle aged man, I was particularly conscious of writing a book which might be of special benefit to other overweight, middle aged men!

I have pulled together an eclectic mix of everything I've learnt about getting things done. It might also help you to know that:

- I'm British, and I have adopted London as my home.
- Across the London Tech Community I'm known as Proactive Paul.
- I'm a qualified first aider.
- I'm a qualified lifeguard.
- I'm a qualified school teacher.
- I'm a qualified accountant.
- I'm proficient in two foreign languages, speak three others, and failed to cope learning three more.
- I'm a professional speaker, mainly in English, and sometimes in French or in Japanese.
- I'm an author of several non-fiction books.
- I spend a lot of time in Japan and have adopted Fukuoka as my home from home.

Across all of these roles I have learnt a lot. It's all channelled in one specific direction. To help you to complete a marathon without going through as much pain, and anguish, and heartache as I did. Excepting a few inevitable set backs, my journey has largely been a series of successive, small wins. Each one building on the foundations of the previous ones. Each one contributing to the positive self reinforcing feedback loop.

Along the way there have been dozens of luminaries who have helped me. They are all detailed in the Bibliography. I read widely, and I take inspiration from a diverse array of seemingly unrelated material. Among them is René Descartes who in 1637 advised:

> *"it is everyone's duty to benefit their fellow men if they can"*

Men, and women, and non-binaries, I would like to help all of you improve your health and fitness. Please take your time, read this book in full, and I hope it gives you a head start so that you'll be better prepared than I was.

Prepared for the challenge of your first, your second, and your third marathon.

Chapter 1 - What exactly are you trying to do?

Chucking Spears

The audience listened carefully as Steve Backley gave a detailed explanation of how he came to discover that he was "pretty good at chucking spears".

Twenty years ago, when the local Chamber of Commerce was a force to be reckoned with, my young, immature business was growing and it was in need of a boost and a few more customers. In order to help improve things, I had acquired the habit of attending regular face to face meetings and events, aiming to make connections, and to learn more about running a successful business. When I discovered that Steve Backley was scheduled to deliver a business talk entitled "The Champion in All of Us" I simply had to go.

There were three reasons. Not only was I making business connections, I was also learning more about how to run a successful business of my own, and thirdly, I was hoping to learn something about improving my own personal health and fitness by finding out more about Steve's journey.

One year earlier, on 1 May 2005 I had joined a local gym. Succumbing to the Bank Holiday promotion of "50% off for the first three months" I paid the discounted fee. And as directed, I and a few other new members dutifully arrived (on May Day itself) for the compulsory induction session, which I describe a little further on.

A year later, on 11 May 2006, "The Champion in All of Us" at the Brands Hatch Conference Centre was designed to show us how we can borrow ideas from success in sport in order to make our businesses better. Before the expression had even been invented, Steve was there explaining "transferable skills" to us. I was fascinated by that, and also by the entertaining explanations of his sporting career.

John Backley in his younger days was a budding athlete with a good measure of success. He wanted his son Steve to start running at an early age. So John had entered Steve into the Bexley Heath under 13 cross country race. The thing is, Steve was only eight years old at the time! The story went a bit like this:

Before the race, dad took Steve to one side for a pep talk. "Son, you only have to beat one person today. Just one. And I'll tell you who that is. The last person! Hang on to him all the way round, and just before the finish, sprint past him!"

That was "hang on" in the metaphorical sense, not the literal sense! And that's how eight year old Steve Backley started out as an athlete. Second from last in the Bexley Heath under 13 race. He ran more races, time after time, until about the age of 12. Then he was involved in an accident which put an end to his running ambitions. After making a good recovery he learnt that middle distance running proved impossible, but short distances were OK. Although he really wasn't cut out to be a sprinter.

Hence, a young Steve Backley tried out various other track and field events, and he was pleasantly surprised to find out that (in his words) he was "pretty good at chucking spears". Very good, as it turns out. He won three silver medals at three consecutive Olympic Games. Plus a handful of gold medals at other international events.

What Steve also taught me is that athletes using "visioning". They picture themselves crossing the finish line first, or throwing the javelin furthest, and they "vision" the medal being placed around their neck. Each event is planned and visioned, from walking out of the dressing room onto the track, through every step of the performance itself, to acknowledging the cheering crowd at the end.

Plans lead to results. Results lead to satisfaction. And in the case of sporting endeavour, plans lead to better physical and mental wellbeing.

Wellbeing

In 2005 my gym membership was short lived. It's a shame that my own sporting endeavour plan had led to a bit of instant oppression right at start!

There I was, a rotund (but not particularly fat) middle aged man, revisiting a fractious relationship with running. In my school days, and in my twenties and thirties, I had done some running on an off, but nothing serious. I had done enough to know that I didn't like running on grass, whether smooth or rough. Nor on gravel tracks. My periodic bouts of enthusiasm involved running mainly on nicely prepared hard surfaces. My ideal surface (I imagined) would be a perfectly smooth race track like Brands Hatch, but any half decent bit of pavement or road was fine.

Until I joined the gym I had never used a running machine or a treadmill. On day one I went through an oppressive induction and endured the overzealous instruction on how to use all the gym's specialist equipment. Even the equipment which I had no intention of ever touching. I was assigned a "coach" and I was given a paper log sheet. The log was to be collected and returned to reception on every visit. The gym also had a swimming pool, which I used a lot. I used the treadmill regularly, and I sometimes spent time on the exercise bike. After fleeting encounters with various machines which (allegedly) improved my muscle strength, I settled into a weekly indoor routine with a mix of swimming, running on a treadmill, and a bit of cycling on the exercise bike. My log shows that on 1 May 2005 I ran 2.1 miles on a treadmill and it took me 24 mins 40 secs.

At that stage I had no idea that I would do many 10k races, let alone a few half marathons, and three full marathons. My original goal was to lose weight. I saw "exercise" and "gym membership" as a step in the right direction. If I was being generous I could have described my early sporting endeavour plan as "woolly" because there was no real plan, merely a dream.

Over the past twenty years, my fitness plan and my business plan have both morphed. How did I get here? How did *you* get here? How did *you* end up reading this book about running?

Paul Brannigan

Nowadays I'm a business coach. OK, I'm also an amateur runner. There's some overlap between my job and my hobby, but my job is basically to help small businesses make more profit in less time. Is that something that you'd be interest in?

My hobby and my job often involve the same sort of strategies, questions, advice, and planning. I asked you "how did you get here?" and I don't actually need you to tell me the answer. I need you to tell yourself. I tell my clients that I don't have all the answers, you have all the answers. They are somewhere deep inside you. I have all the questions, and it's my job to help you find all your answers no matter how deeply they might be hidden. My super power is asking awkward questions. My other super power is not accepting feeble answers.

Chuck Close

And this is where Chuck Close comes in. Chuck Close was an American artist with an unusual style. More importantly, on account of a single thought provoking quote he has influenced many people within his field and beyond:

"The advice I'd like to give to young artists, or anybody really who'll listen to me, is not to wait around for inspiration.

Inspiration is for amateurs; the rest of us just show up and get to work. If you wait around for the clouds to part and a bolt of lightning to strike you in the brain, you are not going to make an awful lot of work. All the best ideas come out of the process; they come out of the work itself. Things occur to you.

If you're sitting around trying to dream up a great art idea, you can sit there a long time before anything happens. But if you just get to work, something will occur to you and something else that you reject will push you in another direction.

Inspiration is absolutely unnecessary and somehow deceptive. You may feel like you need this great idea before you can get down to work, and I find that's almost never the case."

I use that quote all the time, to inspire me to run, to write my books, and to inspire my business clients to actually start *writing* a business plan!

To get the most from this book (assuming you're a runner) you will need to *write* some things down. If you're sitting around trying to write something deep, or profound, you can sit there a long time before anything happens. But if you just start, something will occur to you, write it down, it's for you, not for anybody else, just get it down on paper. You can modify it later, something that you reject will push you in another direction, just write down whatever comes to mind!

Handwriting

And one more thing. This is me, paraphrasing multiple authors, paraphrasing Benjamin Franklin:

"The best way to get things done is almost always to make a plan . . . and more specifically, to write down your plan."

Research has shown that visually mapping out your thoughts by *writing* engages the mind more than *typing*. This leaves you feeling more connected to your material. The frontal lobe of the brain, which is responsible for writing, also controls planning and problem solving. Just the simple act of handwriting your aims brings you closer to implementing them. Typing up your notes later, in some sort of digital system (on a Zoho wiki or Obsidian or Notion, etc), will ensure that you always have access to your notes from any internet connected device. Moreover, hand writing them first and typing them up afterwards is a positive, self reinforcing feedback loop which cements in your mind what you originally wrote down.

The Log

For much of my life, and for many reasons, I have maintained a log. I still have my original glider pilot's log book from the 1970s, and it's wonderful to be able to look back and see the progress from first "air experience flight" aged 14 to flying solo for the first time aged 18.

I recommend that you keep a log, and keep it digitally. The paper log at the gym was abandoned after I quit, which is a shame because it detailed each activity precisely. I also maintained a simple spreadsheet with a summary of my running. That has ten entries over ten weeks in the middle of 2005, and it shows that I gave up on the gym on 10 Jul 2005. I had done 4.2 miles on the treadmill that day. Then there was a big gap until May 2006. Four days after I had met Steve Backley I started running again. Well done Steve, thanks for rekindling the flame! On 15 May 2006 I went for a short 1.5 mile run. Better than nothing!

In 2007 I started maintaining a private wiki for brainstorming, for logging all my races and for recording personal bests. A wiki is a flexible website, it's explained more in Chapter 2 and there's an example at Appendix 3.

There's a page on my wiki for an injury log, and other pages for my personal catalogue of running routes, spanning several major cities and towns across the UK. There are also pages for my routes in Ireland, France, Switzerland and Japan. Nowadays, even when I'm on holiday, I generally stick to my customary routine of running three times per week.

It's wonderful to be able to look back and see how my performance has improved. I know my distance, time, weight, and blood pressure on exactly 1 May 2005. I can see many peaks and troughs over the years. The overall trend is demonstrably positive, and evidenced in the log and supported by some public records for the official races I've entered.

The quality of the running log has improved over time, it has acquired a few more column headings, including one for "notes". It's on a spreadsheet, so that it's searchable, and I can find anything within seconds . . . as long as I actually wrote it down!

I didn't start maintaining a separate injury log until 15 Jul 2012 when I had serious trouble with a pulled muscle. Of all the places it could have been, that was unexpectedly in my shoulder! There's more about that later in the book.

You will find that as you get older, a running log and an injury log are a tremendous help in telling you your own limitations. Your younger self should get into the habit of writing advice and recommendations for your older self. Your older self will regularly thank your younger self for having done that well. It's also refreshing to see how time and distance, and maybe weight and blood pressure change over time. As of the date of publication of this book, November 2024, I am lighter than I have been at any time in the past twenty years.

One day, when I eventually give up running, I will still have the log. I will have reliable, accurate information to share with my children and my grandchildren.

I recommend that you keep a log! A valuable and satisfying tool which helps improve your physical and mental wellbeing. Even when the entries look flaky they serve as motivation. They make you think "come on, you really need to get out and work on that again".

Confucius

It all comes down to a question of discipline. There's a meme, with humorous intent, which you can sometimes find on social media:

> *"Running is nothing more than a series of arguments between the part of your brain that wants to stop and the part that wants to keep going."*

I don't have an attribution for that one. However, we are reliably informed that Confucius did say something like:

> *"Discipline is just choosing between what you want now and want you want most."*

What do you want most? High up on my agenda is a long, healthy life. In order to achieve that I find that running, and weight management, and a disciplined diet help. I have never followed a formal diet, but I've adapted my natural diet. I am not a natural runner, but I've become a pragmatic runner. In my experience running and diet give rise automatically and effectively to good weight control. And if we believe much of the material we are presented with these days, then I have also reduced the risk of contracting many of the so called lifestyle diseases. Whilst I have the physical and mental capacity to continue I plan to maintain this disciplined lifestyle.

Your Task

Before you go on to Chapter 2 you have some homework to do. I'm asking you to follow Chuck Close's advice and just write something down. Nobody will judge you. Nobody else needs to see it. I want you to write it for you.

Starting now.

Grab a pen and a sheet of paper, and write down the answers to the questions at the top of the next page:

1. How did you get here?
2. How did you end up reading this book about running?
3. Why?
4. What are you hoping to achieve?
5. Where does it all end?
6. When you get to the end of this new self imposed plan, how will you know if it's been a good experience?

Kick these ideas around a bit, refine your scribbly notes, modify them. Adapt the questions if you really want to, merge bits, add other bits. Something that you reject will push you in another direction, just write down whatever comes to mind! One of the strategies that business coaches and amateur runners share is writing things down.

Be brave! You can do it! Something that fills a single sheet of A4 is plenty, half a sheet of A4 is enough.

Do that now, before you go on to Chapter 2. Thank you.

Early in Chapter 2 you will also learn about my own answer to the question:

"What exactly are you trying to do?"

Chapter 2 - Everything you need to get started

What, Why and How

When is the best time to take up running?

When you have some passion! Any passion. About anything relevant. It doesn't have to be passion for running. I was passionate about putting my life in order. Seventh wedding anniversary behind me, a four year old child about to start school, my weight was bordering on obese, and I had a number of bad habits that I could do without.

I was passionate about being fit, being healthy, being a good husband, being a good dad, and living a long and fulfilling life. The sub title of this book makes it clear - the objective is to live longer not to kill yourself! Moreover, for somebody with too many outgoings and not enough income, I needed something which could fit into the centre of a Venn diagram like this:

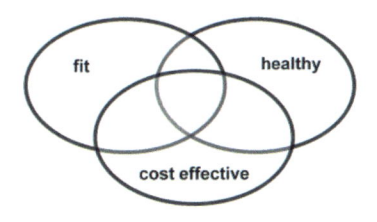

Running is (in theory) a cheap hobby.

You might look at the Venn diagram and instinctively come up with something else. In my case the gut feeling and the immediate thought was "running". In these situations psychologists may tell you that the first thing that comes into your head is probably the right answer. Although the magic word was "running" I didn't wholly buy into that at first. I mentioned before that I had done a modest amount of running when I was younger. However, the word "running" kept coming back to haunt me, and eventually the plan and the Venn diagram both coalesced around this particular word.

The best time to take up running is when your passion and objectives all line up and point to "running" as the best all-round course of action. And then you'll do it. Not running for the sake of running. Running for the sake of your own sanity and quality of life. That's why I do it. Every time I finish I get a dopamine rush. Mild, moderate or massive. Every time. Dopamine is the happy hormone, you get it from exercising, from cooking, and from listening to music, and it helps boost your feel-good factor. I get lots of it, especially when I run and also when I swim.

It took me a long time before I settled into a regular, repetitive, happy routine. The current routine sees me in the right running kit, with the right shoes, going out three times per week, doing a variety of routes and distances, on level paved surfaces, with minimal ascents and descents.

My routine starts and ends at my front door, not at the gym. That means it's cheap!

It took years of trial and error before I worked out what was right for me. You'll probably have a bit of trial and error yourself. I hope this book leads you to find your happy place in less time than my early misadventures.

At the end of Chapter One I asked you to write down a few things. So did Chuck Close. So I'm assuming that you did write stuff. If you did, and only if you did, you may now see my version of "what exactly are you trying to do, why, how, etc" which is set out for your amusement at Appendix 1. No cheating! Write yours first!

Running Kit

There's a lot of discussion coming up (over two chapters) about running kit, what I chose, how and why I chose it, and sometimes what I abandoned and why. These are all personal preferences and they are shared with you not because they are right or wrong. It's simply what I experienced. Some of my personal preferences might be a bit picky, sorry, we're all human! I would also love to tell you all about the right female clothing, but I'm not able to. Some of the following comment is universal, some of it depends on gender, nonetheless all of my "buying experiences" are set out below to help everybody.

There is some meticulous detail in these chapters, and although I have a good memory, it's largely because I maintain a log. If I have good or bad experiences with something, especially with shoes, I make notes that day. How, where, why, what. I don't want to make the same mistake twice, so my younger self writes notes for my older self. That's a good habit to get into.

Once I have a system or a product that works for me I stick with it. When it comes to clothing, I have no doubt I could improve more, but when I've found something that works nicely for me I'm not willing to spend more money experimenting with new variations of kit.

Bear in mind that I'm not strictly a "running enthusiast". I'm an advocate of being fit and healthy, and it just happens to be the case that *running* fits my agenda. I am also prepared to spend a sensible amount of money on sensible kit. However, I will not spend more than I judge to be about right. My running shoes are a bit upmarket, my other kit is value for money stuff. If the running top is well priced with suitably thin, breathable material, and the logo is weird, I will still buy it. I do not need to spend more on perfect attire.

Initially it came as a surprise to me that some of the stuff I bought didn't work out the way I expected, so I discarded it. I'm a little fussy about my running kit, and even more fussy about some of the businesses and the brands that sell it. There are no recommendations to use or avoid certain brands. Some opinions will inevitably emerge, but I shall try to keep it factual, and help the amateur runners who are reading this.

You don't need any special running kit to go out today and start running. The more distance you cover, and the longer your duration, the more likely you are to begin to want to assemble the right kit for you, especially the right shoes! It might take a bit of time and money to get things right in the shoe department.

Shoes

Wearing whatever daytime clothing you normally wear, you can run for the bus! You can start running short distances with anything you have. Any old trainers, shorts and T shirt will do. Tracksuit if you prefer, or any old long sleeve top. The shoes are important, worn in, but not worn out, and probably not brand new. New shoes need to worn a couple of times, before you use them for really serious running.

The cheapest trainers from the cheapest shops are best avoided, in the same way that cheap everyday shoes are doing your feet no favours. Lift the insole inside your shoe, any shoe, and have a look below it. Is the sole a continuous solid mass or does it resemble a honeycomb or lattice work waffle? One which has a large expanse of holes and a few ridges? Those ridges will lead to injuries.

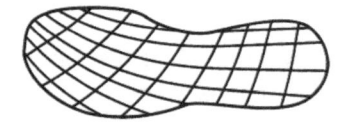

Avoid shoes with hidden, internal lattice work

Shoes in general

Once upon a time when I was a penniless youngster I had the cheapest business style brogues I could find. I wore them to work every day. When I went to the clinic my GP instructed me to remove one shoe, lift the insole, and then he showed me the lattice work. And he explained that this was the precise reason for the pinch points and the pain on the soles of my feet. Half a dozen ridges biting into the heel of my foot while 80% of the surface area was nothing but air.

Trainers

Throughout my teenage years, through my twenties and thirties I had used decent, ordinary trainers for all my sporting activities, and that included a bit of road running. I had no particular brand loyalty, though I did tend to stick with reputable stuff like Reebok or Adidas. My casual clothing has (for many years) included Reebok DMX Ride Advanced 3.0 trainers. I buy them at Lillywhites on Piccadilly Circus, usually in the January sales, and usually two pairs at a time.

In the Gym, way back in 2005/6, I used those ordinary Reebok trainers on the treadmill. Until the coach, aware that some of us had entered the local 10k race, decided that we should get out on the road and do some real running. The gym added outdoor running sessions to the timetable, and established a 5k route.

Oh my word! Road! The trouble with running on a road is that it does not automatically progress in a speedy fashion beneath your feet. Not like a treadmill. Oh no, you actually have to run! And move your own body weight in a purposeful fashion without any electrical assistance! After two or three of those outdoor sessions I gave up using the treadmill. What's the point? It is honestly nothing like running in real life.

Maybe I'm being a bit harsh? Training on treadmills is better than nothing, but it's nothing like running on a road!

Running shoes

A couple of weeks passed, several outdoor sessions passed, and then one of the coaches noticed my favourite Reebok trainers.

"You'll need proper running shoes you know!"

"I will? I mean . . . I will!"

Seriously? I need proper running shoes? That's more expense on top of gym membership, and I was a bit suspicious of the way his dialogue developed. Go down to the stadium (the one where the 10k was scheduled to start later that year) visit the professional shop and get a running assessment done. Somewhat reluctantly I did as I was told. Not because I trusted the coach, but more because my curiosity had been aroused, and I wanted to know what this free video based running assessment was all about. And why hadn't I been told this in the gym two weeks earlier, when the road running group was first assembled?

A pleasant lady answered the shop's phone (those were the days, robot phone systems hadn't yet been invented) and I booked a 30 minute slot for my free assessment. As a complete novice runner (I might as well have had the word "gullible" written across my forehead as I walked through the door) I followed the procedure exactly as directed. I ran on a treadmill. I watched the video of the gait analysis. What's so special about all of this I thought? My running looked quite normal to me, if a bit slow. I was told that I pronate very slightly. I faked a sincere nod of acquiescence, which the pleasant lady had no doubt recognised as a *fake* sincere nod of acquiescence. And she set up me up for the sale by saying that the pronation was insignificant and that no adjustment (no inserts) would be needed for proper professional running shoes . . . like these ones . . . at only *megabucks*.

Ordinarily I wear UK size 7 shoes, or size 7.5 if I can find them. But it's not easy finding half sizes for my everyday professional shoes or my everyday trainers. This sports shop didn't stock half sizes either, and had insisted that my running shoes therefore needed to be size 8. That's what I bought. Especially as I had been told to buy cushioned socks as well.

I don't have an exact figure, but as I recall the shoes cost about £60. That was about twice what I would normally have spent on decent Reebok or Adidas trainers. To be honest, I thought the running shoes were expensive, but that wasn't life threatening amounts of money, and it was certainly a lot cheaper than many of the sets of elite shoes dotted around the shop. I went home unsure if I was the proud new owner (or just a gullible new owner) of the current model of lurid blue New Balance 560 Tech Ride running shoes.

The New Balance shoes were fine, proper running shoes, neither elite nor basic, and they were probably about right for what I needed at the time. I was never 100% happy with the fit, but they did the job and I clocked up the miles. In the early days, my log recorded distances in miles, even though I was training for a 10 kilometre race. The shoes are designed with a soft sole which wears out over time. The recommendation is to replace running shoes at 500 miles, or when the surface of the sole wears out (and the "other colour" begins to show), whichever comes sooner.

I made a point of using my expensive shoes until about 750 miles. I'm not an elite runner, not even a competitive runner, just an amateur. Even though the sole was visibly worn, I could feel no difference in the shoe at 1 mile or at 750 miles. Anyway, the shoes were changed after 750 miles. The fun and games of getting the right shoes is a never ending story. Running shoes are probably the most important piece of kit you will buy, and my experiences with more and more shoes take up the whole of the next chapter.

Socks and Pants

Not too far from where I live there is a big retail park with a number of major brands. These outlets have a reputation for offering some end of line products at cheaper prices than normal stores. From the Sports Direct shop I bought ankle length white socks with a cushioned base. They made no difference to me, certainly not physically. Psychologically I wanted to feel that I had made the right decision. But psychologically I wasn't convinced either. I used them until they wore out and I never bought cushioned socks again.

For a long time I stuck with the same simple, cheap, plain white sports socks, as I had always done. That's what I was wearing when I was sold the New Balance shoes. The new fangled cushioned socks were bought a day or two later, and I never really felt comfortable with them. We're probably talking only about one millimetre or less, but I was used to simple socks, I had run in simple socks for decades, and (excepting a bit of 2005/6 with cushioned socks) plain socks are what I use to this day. I've also given up buying white socks. My daily attire merits black socks, and so that's all I buy now. And I use them for everything, including running. It's what I feel most comfortable with, and comfort is key when I run. A nicely fitted sock in a nicely fitted shoe. Physically comfortable and psychologically right. Purists and competitive runners may look on aghast! But I'm an amateur runner and having tried to do the cushioned sock thing, I now prefer to do my own thing.

And what about pants? I mean "underwear" in case any Americans are reading this. My regular attire back then was the classic polyester cotton slip. From Marks & Spencer or John Lewis I think. Slightly better quality than the ones you could get in a big Sainsbury or Tesco store, but nothing extravagant. I wore them all day, every day, for work, rest and play. They were fine for running, so I used them when I ran. Nothing to report really! Just bog standard polyester cotton slips at posh store prices.

Until a bit later! With age and experience, my income and my lifestyle improved. Long after my early racing exploits I learnt about the merits of 100% cotton underwear, and I started buying slips with this higher spec material. Still the classic slip style, but better quality. It's a material that holds on to sweat longer, and a material that becomes more uncomfortable the longer you run. During my training for my second marathon I learnt that 100% cotton underwear is not suitable for running. I started running commando. I ran the Geneva Marathon in loose fitting shorts with no underwear. In my book *comfort* rules!

Running commando didn't trouble me, but I was advised by other runners to get some specialist running pants. The keen runners all told me to buy Runderwear. They're a bit pricey, but I was willing to try them, especially as they are close fitting slips. I bought one twin pack and tried them out for running.

First impression, putting them on, incredibly comfortable. Made from 92% polyamide and 8% elastane they are 100% synthetic. Yet they are far superior to the polyester cotton I had used in the past. Hopefully they fit the bill in the same way? Yes and no. They are certainly OK for running, but after years of running commando I was used to that. I bought some more Runderwear. Sometimes I would wear them to run, sometimes not. I gave them a fair chance. They are nice, and they are probably worth paying more for. They are now my everyday pants. No more 100% cotton. However, I still prefer to run commando. No underwear when running, and Runderwear when not running. Feel free to point and laugh at me!

What do the ladies wear? Anecdotally, I have heard that Runderwear is the leading brand for ladies too. However, I don't know. I'm an old man who has refrained from asking the ladies intimate questions about their choice of underwear. The female runners in central London are predominantly *young* ladies. You might be in a better position to ask them than me. I shall continue to avoid any risk of being labelled a dirty old man!

Shorts and T Shirts

Close fitting, or baggy, or somewhere between the two?

My early experiences of running (in the 1970s and 1980s) were coloured by TV images of handsome young men with fashionable clothing and an enviable physique. John Travolta in Saturday Night Fever, Steve Austin the Six Million Dollar Man, and others of that genre from the late 1970s. My close fitting shorts and skimpy running vests certainly showed off my less than perfect physique, and they did absolutely nothing for my macho appeal.

By 2005 I was carrying more fat, and I took to wearing running gear which was one size bigger than normal for a chap of medium height and build. I had the perennial problem of size, what one brand calls M, another brand labels as L.

My wife tells me that ladies dresses vary from shop to shop. Well menswear does too. For the first time in my life I started wearing XL or XXL T shirts and shorts. Partly, because I was overweight, and partly because anything smaller became uncomfortable when it was wet with sweat. I worked hard at my exercise routines, and I learnt that I sweat profusely.

Over time, I moved from everyday, cheap polyester cotton T shirts, to a brief relationship with 100% cotton ones, before settling on fully synthetic wicking shirts for runners. The brand I use is AWD (All We Do) and that's what you can see me wearing in the cover photo. Now that I've established a preferred T shirt I simply reorder the same thing on Amazon. I have been doing this for years, because almost none of the retail shops will sell me the "same thing I had last time".

At size XXL, my T shirts are one size too big. Now that I've lost weight they are probably two sizes too big. I stuck with them right up to mid 2024.

The same goes for shorts. My shorts are way too big. The cover photo shows me wearing plain black football shorts. They are size XXL and when I'm standing still the legs of these shorts reach just below my knees. Ideal for me when I ran, plenty of space, lots of air circulation, and fewer problems with sweat.

They are 100% polyester and are described as Jogging Running Football Gym Breathable Sports Shorts. Or in my vernacular, High Rise Football Shorts.

Outer wear

As the cover shows you, I also wear a sweatband on my head. Bjorn Borg wore one at Wimbledon. So it's OK. Mark Knopfler wears one to play guitar! So it's OK. I wear one because my head sweats industrial grade hydrochloric acid, and it stings like mad when it runs into my eyes!

I'm not fussy about outer wear. A simple and cheap terylene sweatband is my philosophy here. They come from somewhere in China, and I buy them three at a time, on eBay. Never finding the same supplier twice, but almost always getting the exact same product every time.

Lillywhites provides me with other handy items. My wiki tells me that the last time I bought them (on 2 January 2018) I had:

- Karrimor Xlite Lightweight Jacket Fluo Yellow (Medium) reduced from £53.99 to £13.99
- Karrimor Running Gloves reduced from £9.99 to £4.99

I want them to keep the wind at bay. They're not much good against persistent rain, but they take the edge off a cutting wind.

Up the road from Piccadilly Circus, on Regent Street proper, there is a Uniqlo store where I normally buy simple, tracksuit trousers. The pair that I bought recently, at a Uniqlo store in Japan on 17 Sep 2023 cost me ¥2,290 (roughly £12.50), about half of what I would have paid in London!

For warmth on colder runs I have a lightweight long sleeved top. I prefer many layers of thin clothes, so that I can remove one layer if needed. When I did my training in Geneva over the cold winter of 2017/18 the temperature could be as low as minus 9°C. I still went out, I would wear the dayglo jacket, over two layers of long sleeve tops, over one T shirt. That winter was the only time I wore two long sleeve tops on training runs. It was also the only time I ever wore a woolly hat to run, and it was the only time I ever ran on snow.

My long sleeve tops vary over the years, depending on what I can get. Currently they are "Killer Whale Running Top Mens Long Sleeve T Shirt Light Weight UPF 50". I don't like the logo nor the brand name, but it's exactly the right attire for me, the correct thickness (thinness) and price. I have three of them at size XL and they cost me £17.00 a time.

Finally, I have a cheap white baseball cap, also from a Chinese vendor on eBay. I wear it in bright sunshine (that's rare) and when it rains (that's more common). Baseball caps are not my thing, and you'd never normally see me wearing one. However when I run, a baseball cap is perfect for keeping the sun out of my eyes, and for keeping 99% of raindrops off my glasses. The cap is adjustable and fits nicely over the sweat band. When the cap is not needed it's returned to a large external pocket on the back of my runners backpack. The pocket is arranged so that I can remove and replace the cap while still running.

Bum Bag

For many years, I used a simple bum bag to carry assorted goodies like my keys, phone, one bank card, and a little cash. Enough to get me out of emergencies, and enough (if I became unconscious) for my rescuer to know my name. It was also big enough to carry one or two disposable pouches for water. The bum bag is slightly awkward to run with, but it's something you quickly learn to accommodate.

Runners Backpack

After a friend of mine at the Geneva Runners Club gave me a thorough introduction to his expensive, fancy backpack, I was convinced it was a far better solution than a bum bag, and it had the added bonus that it could carry 1.5 litres of water. That's more than enough to get me through a half marathon.

From Amazon I bought the Aonijie 5 litre backpack (5 litres of total storage, not water storage) for £20.99, because it has a vast array of small pockets. Variously I use the pockets to store:

iPhone	bank card	gloves
ten quid	keys	energy source (sweets/gel)
driving licence	lip salve	baseball cap

That leaves enough space for me to cram in either a plastic pac-a-mac, or a lightweight long sleeve top. The straps are a bit fussy, and can become loose. The ones at the sides have now been stapled together to keep them at the correct length, and gaffer tape has been wrapped around that, to stop the ends of the staples from stabbing me!

I also carry a tiny, thin cotton towel, draped over the top strap, so that I can easily take it to wipe away sweat, and put in back in place again. It vaguely looks like I'm wearing a baby's bib. The utility of my sweat rag outweighs the minor eccentricity in my appearance.

The original 1.5 litre water bladder was a bit fussy (with a slider device to seal the top) and I have replaced it with a sturdier one (with a large circular screw cap). No matter what the spiel says about "leak proof" your bladder will wear out and leak! Sometimes after a few weeks, sometimes after a few months.

My strategy is to repair the leak in the same way that I repair a bicycle inner tube. A small patch from a puncture repair kit does the job. Left overnight, the patch becomes secure, and then I use one loop of gaffer tape to fully encircle the bladder over the patched area. The gaffer tape keeps the edges of the patch from chafing on the fabric of the backpack.

The repair will certainly last a week, usually more, and that's long enough to order and receive a replacement bladder.

When the new bladder arrives, check how the pipe is fitted to the base.

The screw fit version is far superior. The push fit one with a release tab is less secure, there will be seepage, and air will find its way into the bladder. That leads to an air pocket forming at the top, which leads to an irritating noise if you try to run with the sound of water sloshing around right behind your head

Backpack
www.dontreadmyblog.com

More notes (and photos) of my modified backpack are included in a blogpost on my website.

Rainwear

What happens if it rains?

You get wet!

I've done several training runs in the rain. I have done two half marathons in the rain. Fortunately, there was no rain when I completed each of my full marathons. There's more detail on inclement weather in Chapters 6 and 10.

Sundry

There are a few other things that help, although they may not need to be carried on you when you run. Variously I use things like sun block and a moisturiser cream before I run. These are listed on a "daily routine" checklist which I work through before I go out on a morning run.

My checklist also says "expel air", because when you leave the same water in the bladder for 48 hours, there's a risk that there might be more air in the bladder. If it starts sloshing around I'm not going to stop running at about the 100m point and expel it. Hence, I routinely do it before I run.

A checklist might help you too. Add your own personal notes to your checklist. Plan to help your older self understand *how* and *why* you do what you do.

Comfort

Once you're comfortable with your kit and your routine you'll have fewer things to worry about. Learn quickly, and you'll spend less money too!

Advance preparation leads to improved peace of mind.

Chapter 3 - Shoes, Shoes and More Shoes

Comfort

In 490BC when he ran barefoot from Marathon to Athens, Pheidippides probably didn't have to contend with broken glass bottles and the other detritus of 21st century city life.

How important are shoes? Do you even need shoes?

I'm not going to discuss the detail of barefoot running, but the British Medical Journal did, in an article in 2020, and they found some evidence that modern running shoes have led to a small *increase* in reported injuries! However, given that running has developed from a popular past time back in the 1970s, to a big business nowadays, I think the increased number of enthusiasts may explain the *increase* in reported injuries. The BMJ also stresses that large changes to our footwear habits have occurred in a very short space of time relative to the evolution of the human species. Humans may not have adapted as fast as the footwear manufacturers have. The authors of the BMJ article seem to cautiously like the concept of barefoot running, and make recommendations about how runners might do that in a modern urban environment.

I use shoes.

My journey has been long and costly. It's here, warts and all, so that you can see what you might be letting yourself in for. Like the last chapter, this chapter is full of my personal opinions, based on my experiences. My opinions are neither right nor wrong. They are simply about what is right for me. The choices I've made normally help my physical health and my mental health. I'm not into analysing running habits to the Nth degree. I just need to be somewhere comfortable with my own habits.

None of this dialogue amounts to a recommendation.

Adidas or Reebok

Until I was 44 years old I used to run with whatever trainers I happened to own. Generally they came from Adidas or Reebok. My old photographs tell me that I used Adidas in my teens and early twenties, and by my mid thirties I had adopted Reebok. Reebok is my wife's favourite. None of these shoes were anything special, certainly not expensive, but they were better than the cheap, basic things that I could have bought in larger supermarkets. Pleasant, general purpose trainers, and they caused me no problems and no injuries.

New Balance 560 Tech Ride - Approx 31 May 2005 - Approx £60.00

To be honest, I had never heard of New Balance until the day that I bought these shoes.

I'm a creature of habit. Once I find some sort of clothing that I like, I want to buy the same thing over and over again. Clarks leather shoes for one thing, and other types of sober, formal business wear. When I can't get the same type of shirt as last time, I really get quite upset with John Lewis.

Hence, these new lurid blue New Balance 560 Tech Ride running shoes which I bought in 2006 took some getting used to. I had some misgivings about the way I had been coerced into buying them (see the previous chapter), but I never really suffered buyers' remorse. They were my first pair of proper running shoes and they did the job nicely. I used them for several years and I exceeded the recommended "change them after 500 miles" rule. In that time I had competed countless training runs, several 10k races, and my first two half marathons.

Personally, I worry that the 500 mile rule was invented by shoe manufacturers who want to sell more shoes. When it comes to all of my other footwear, I use them until they wear out and then I replace them. Actually, that tends to happen with my running shoes as well, but not strictly according to the 500 mile rule. You will need to change your running shoes periodically. The point is that the *suppleness* and the *cushioning* deteriorates over time and without that you have more stresses on your legs, and an increased risk of injury. The soles of the shoes tend to have little nodes that wear down first. The ones at the toes and the heel wear down faster and you can compare them to the ones in the arch of the foot. When the wear and tear on some of the nodes makes them level with the base material, then (the manufacturer's say) it's time to change them.

These New Balance 560 Tech Ride shoes became pretty worn out, though I had grown to like them. However, I was wary about keeping "my comfortable, familiar running shoes" for my first marathon in 2013. By which time they would have literally been falling to bits. The question then became "when do I replace them" because the other problem was that I didn't want to be running my first marathon in brand new shoes which had not yet been adequately worn in.

New Balance N2 - 9 Oct 2012 - Special Offer £36.00

Naturally, I wanted the same shoe as last time. I wanted New Balance 560 Tech Ride, and I couldn't find them anywhere! I had to go for the nearest equivalent, and that took a lot of searching.

There were six months to go before my first marathon, I was stepping up the number of training runs, and those runs were becoming progressively longer. If I bought new shoes in October 2012 they would be well worn in by May 2013, but they wouldn't be worn out!

I searched online, and I went to various shops in London. I found my second pair of running shoes in Harrods! No, I don't normally shop in Harrods. During my entire life I think I have bought something there three times! I was in luck though, because in 2012 the Harrods sports department was closing down, to be replaced by another, and they were selling off their stock. The New Balance N2 was a pretty close match with the 560 Tech Ride, and it was reduced. I paid £36.00 instead of the advertised price of £72.00.

All in all, I was pretty pleased with myself. They were comfortable, almost the same as my previous shoe, and they were cheaper in Harrods than they were on Amazon!

They also came in for a lot more mileage a lot quicker than my originals, and they lasted me just four years in contrast to the previous six.

I wanted the same thing again, again!

New Balance M560RB2 - 15 Apr 2017 - Approx £55.00

Whilst on holiday in Japan I found a big, reputable department store with a good sized sports department. And they had the same shoe. It looked like a perfect match for my New Balance N2 which I had brought with me on holiday. I have 10k training routes in my adopted home town in Japan, so I take my running kit on holidays!

The shoes in the shop were not labelled New Balance N2, but New Balance M560RB2, and comparing them side by side, I was certain that they were the same thing. Not wanting to pass up the chance of getting exactly what I wanted (if a few weeks earlier than planned) I bought them for ¥7,560 or £54.23 if you prefer.

Within two months I was finding them uncomfortable. My log tells me that on 28 May 2017 a small blister developed on my left foot.

Blisters happen when there is too much movement of the foot inside the shoe, and that can normally be remedied by wearing thicker socks. You can also try wearing ladies' nylon pop socks under your regular socks. That's enough to achieve zero movement between the skin and the first layer of clothing. It's movement between the skin and the first layer of clothing that causes the blister.

Anyway, checking my log I can see that on 28 May 2017 I wrote "running shoes are causing blisters, because the insole rises at the instep, there is a gap between the shoe wall and insole, and the loose ridge moves". The ridge moved with every stride, repeatedly creating and closing a tiny gap, leading to enough friction to cause a blister.

I was training for my second marathon at the time, and was living in Geneva. Two days later, the entry in my log says "I ran the 10k CERN Loop and ended up with a 40mm blister on my right foot, and chafing on my left" and later added a note "The blister was not fully blown and it dissipated after 2 days".

Three months after I had bought these shoes, on 1 Jul 2017, a hole began to appear. These shoes were the same size as the previous ones, size 8 (or 42) and my big toe was pushing a hole through the upper on the left shoe. It seems that the shoes were loose enough to cause blisters, and tight enough to cause a hole.

It was now the school summer holidays, I was back in London, and I was searching for new running shoes. In spite of my misgivings about professional sports shops I went to one near Victoria Station expecting a repeat of the gait assessment, the video analysis and the dialogue I had been through many years earlier (at a shop in Kent). No treadmill, the gait analysis was done by a staff member watching me run along the pavement outside the shop. No video, but plenty of dialogue. One way dialogue! Please let *me* talk! I had brought my defective shoes with me, and I wanted to explain my concerns and my precise needs. The shop assistant had zero interest in my dialogue, and simply wanted to make a sale. A pretty expensive sale. I left empty handed, on account of her attitude, not on account the high prices, which I would have probably paid if they had the right shoes, and appropriate levels of customer service.

My log for 11 Aug 2017 says "not going back".

A few days later, still using my New Balance shoes there was not just one hole, now the right shoe was giving me gip. On 17 Aug 2017 my log says "a tiny hole has appeared in right shoe where big toe fits - left shoe hole is now 14mm x 5mm - going to Lillywhites tomorrow - sound instep is what I need most".

The thought crossed my mind that these may have been cheap counterfeit copies. If that was the case then "BigCo" (my reputable store in Japan) was probably duped the same way that I was. I have used that store for many things over many years. The shoe originally looked right and felt right in very way. It was six weeks before something minor felt wrong and another six weeks before something major went wrong. What seems especially odd is that the shoes developed holes but there were no corresponding holes in any of my socks!

Either, one of the buyers at "BigCo", or one of the intermediaries in the supply chain had succumbed to the racket of substituting counterfeit goods.

I'm not saying that the problem could be traced back to China. But look up *Pandabuy* and you will see how some of these schemes work. Pandabuy is a shopping agent platform, acting as a link between sellers and buyers. It doesn't manufacture anything, but has become famous as a source of cheap and allegedly fake designer goods. Influencers and customers regularly post videos of their Pandabuy problems on TikTok, Discord, and other social media platforms.

Replacement shoes were needed urgently. I visited Lillywhites on 18 Aug 2017 and I tried on various shoes. Lillywhites has a treadmill, and staff who do not pester you for a sale. I bought a Karrimor lightweight jacket and some Karrimor running gloves, but I did not buy running shoes that day. However, I did like the Nike Air Max Motion priced at £70.00, I just wasn't sure that they were right, and I also had the feeling that they were a bit cheap when most of the running shoes were higher priced.

Discussions with friends followed, and I did a lot of web searches.

Nike Air Zoom Pegasus 34 - 25 Aug 2017 - £99.99

One week later I went back to Lillywhites. Based on a recommendation or two I was aiming to buy Nike Air Pegasus. What I bought was Nike Air Zoom Pegasus 34 in size 7. My formal shoes are size 7, but my running shoes have all been size 8. Using the treadmill in Lillywhites I tried size 8 and size 7.5 and size 7. I was delighted to see that Nike does half sizes and that Lillywhites stocks them. Although the size 7.5 felt a little too big.

The size 7 fitted like a glove. All nice and snug, like close fitting slippers, or ridiculously thick socks. Really comfortable, and as at that date they were the best shoe that I had ever tried on.

Obviously, these running shoes are not exactly like wearing slippers. Nor are they like my regular, professional shoes. Just think of them as being very close to slippers, and nothing like leather shoes.

I was now the proud owner of Nike Air Zoom Pegasus 34 shoes for £99.99. What was even better, is that instead of being lurid blue, these were a nice, sober black. They're the ones in the photo on the cover of this book.

I put miles and miles on them. I ran the Geneva Marathon wearing them. I was happy with them until I reached the marathon's 35k waypoint.

During training for Geneva I had covered 35k a couple of times with no discomfort. However, on marathon day I made a mental note at about 35k that my shoes were feeling tight. By the time I got home it was 4pm. I made more notes in my log, went online and immediately ordered a new pair. Not size 7 this time, but size 7.5.

Nike Air Zoom Pegasus 34 - 6 May 2018 - Approx £73.00

Identical in every respect to the pair that I had tried on in Lillywhites, these new ones were the same sober black, and cost CHF99.99 or £72.97. In spite of being in Switzerland, these were cheaper than my London ones, and they were delivered to my doorstep. I now realised that size 7.5 was what I had really needed all along.

The problem with finding nice shoes that you really like, is that the manufacturer discontinues them and you have to try something new and different.

Nike Air Zoom Pegasus 34 - 22 Jun 2021 - £89.99

In 2021, none of the shops had Nike Air Zoom Pegasus 34 anymore. Nor were they popping up on Amazon much. And certainly not in my size of 7.5. I got into the habit of checking Amazon regularly, on the off chance that some "Market Place" retailer would have them. Bingo! On 22 Jun 2021 I ordered some blue ones for £89.99. I didn't need them just yet, but I wanted them on hand for the day when the replacement became necessary.

My son liked them, and they instantly became his shoes! Yes, he has the same size feet as me.

I never found the same ones again, and I continued using my old black ones until they were completely worn out.

Nike Air Zoom Pegasus 38 - 26 Nov 2021 - £82.02

In late 2021 the latest version of the shoe was a 38 not a 34. And they looked ugly! I bought them for £82.02, tried them on at home, didn't like the feel, didn't like the look, and certainly didn't like the revised lacing system with chunky fabric loops rather than the fine elasticated ones on the older version.

What was especially troubling was the heel. Extending out from the sole at the back of the shoe there is something that looks like the bow of a ship. It makes the shoe longer and uglier, even if it helps professional runners run professionally. Walking up and down through my flat, jogging on the spot, this extra heel just felt all wrong.

I sent them back for a refund.

Nike Air Zoom Pegasus 38 - 29 Jan 2022 - £60.00

A few weeks after my failed encounter with the new Pegasus 38 I really needed new running shoes. I could no longer find anybody with old stock and so I relented and bought the 38 again. This time in a January sale, and this time they were priced at only £60.00.

That was enough to tempt me to swallow my pride, wear ugly big boats, and suffer a £60.00 risk rather than an £82.00 risk! They are size 7.5 and in my preferred colour black.

Trying them on at home I still didn't like them, and I continued to run in my old 34s. Until the old ones truly split at the seams, and then I had to use the 38s.

I was surprised, instead of being the fashion conscious amateur runner (reader, I am rarely fashion conscious) I discovered that the new shoes are actually quite good for running. New 38s are certainly a lot better than old worn out 34s.

Months later, I became quite accustomed to the 38s. Nice for running, and ugly to look at. So I try to focus on running with them and hide them in the cupboard when I'm not running.

Incidentally, when the new Battersea Power Station shopping centre opened, I went for a visit. There's a Nike store. I noticed that the 38 has been upstaged by the 40. I've not looked at Nike recently so I have no idea what number the Pegasus series has reached now. I'm still trying to buy new old stock on Amazon.

The Brooks Glycerin 18 that never happened - 26 Dec 2023 - £96.00

Next up on my list is Brooks Glycerin. I was on the cusp of ordering some Brooks shoes when unexpectedly I found myself on a break due to injury. In December 2023 a pair of Brooks Glycerin 18 in my size 7.5 (only available in white) would have cost me £96.

There was plenty of life left still in my Nike Air Zoom Pegasus 38s, so my next choice of shoe was deferred for a bit.

At the start of 2024, in both Yokohama and in London, I came across sports shops that had Brooks Glycerin shoes on display. The shoes are probably brilliant, but they look cheap. The sole appears to be some sort of spongy plastic and it looks and feels like a disposable plastic water bottle. Cheap plastic like the cheap bargain store shoes I wore as a kid. I'm probably maligning them unjustly, much to the distress of their scientific advisers. But I don't want to be running around with plastic trampolines strapped to my feet, so I won't be buying Brooks.

Nike Air Zoom Pegasus 38 - 9 Jun 2024 - £93.99

I did some calculations involving distance. I had the same dilemma as in 2013. I had grown to like the ugly Nike Air Zoom Pegasus 38, but they were getting a good deal of use. Nowhere near worn out, but given my training program they would have reached "end of life" at just about the time of the Chelmsford Marathon on 13 Oct 2024. Again I was wary about keeping "my comfortable, familiar running shoes" for the marathon as I didn't want them falling to bits. On 9 Jun 2024 after a 20k training run, I ordered some new shoes for £93.99. They are definitely new old stock these days, and having found a pair of 38s in black, and in size 7.5, I wasn't going to pass up the opportunity.

This newer pair were kept to one side until the end of August and saw their first outing on Thursday 29 Aug 2024 when I did a 15k training run. By using them regularly throughout September they would be settled in by the time I attempted the marathon in October. The training programme said that I was going to cover 280k (174 miles) during September, as I prepared for the race. That looked like "comfortably worn in" by my reckoning, and it allowed me time for a contingency if something went astray with the new shoes.

Comfort

There is much talk, rumour and myth spouted in the sports shops and in some running clubs. I have had fleeting connections with two running clubs, but at my slow pace, I find that running is a solo hobby. Everybody assumes that I am some aspiring hard core enthusiast. I am nothing more than a keen novice.

Depending on who you listen to, you might learn that running causes harm and that the right shoes reduce the risk of harm. Well, for 55 years the only running related injury I had was a pulled muscle in my shoulder. A bit of over enthusiasm with my pre run stretches seems to have caused that pain. Not the running itself.

Later in the book you will read about two lower limb injuries. Both of them were caused by striking an object in the dark.

Running before dawn, on uneven surfaces, led to each injury. Given the condition of the surfaces across much of central London, it could happen to anyone at any speed. A raised manhole cover caused one, and a sunken paving stone caused the other. I no longer run during the hours of darkness, and since taking that decision, I've had no injuries.

Running properly does not cause injuries.
Hitting things unexpectedly, and at awkward angles, causes injuries.

Some studies even conclude that your choice of running shoe demonstrates no reduction in lower limb injuries in adults. Your training load, technique, and muscle strength can influence your susceptibility to injury. My load is graduated, my technique is slow, my habit is methodical running on good surfaces in daylight, and my muscle strength is aided by the exercises I've outline in Chapter 5.

Above all, comfort is key. It's OK to not be OK. If it hurts, stop! If the clothes are not right, experiment until you find something you like. And the same goes for shoes. Nobody can do that journey for you. Like me, you just have to go through trial and error, and when you find something comfortable stick with it. It will take a bit of time, and a bit of money. I've shared my experiences with you so that you can get a good feel for what that journey looks like. Choose shoes that feel good on your feet, and which match your intended terrain.

Should you change your running shoes after 500 miles? You should change them when you feel they have outlived their useful life. Ignore the corporate message about coloured layers on the sole wearing through, and about the nodes being worn down to nothing. Look at the sole and make your own judgement call about when they are genuinely worn out and/or not fit for purpose.

If the sole is badly distressed, or the shoe just feels uncomfortable at any time, change them. My New Balance M560RB2 were binned after just four months due to discomfort. Whereas in the early days, I maxed out every pair of Nike Air Zoom Pegasus 34 I ever had, up until the point where the threads were failing and the joints were just beginning to separate. The soles were still serviceable after the uppers had perished!

The Fold Test

If you're tempted to run with cheaper shoes, just bear in mind that you need supple, cushioned shoes. Do the *fold test* on the shoes in the shop. You should be able to bend running shoes completely in half. You can do that with the better quality shoes like the Nike Air Zoom Pegasus. You don't have to buy Nike Air Zoom Pegasus, but if the shop has them, fold one, and you'll see what I mean.

Pricing

You'll have noticed from the figures above that the price of running shoes appears to lag behind inflation. These days they certainly feel less expensive than they were a few years ago.

Then again, my overall spending on shoes has probably been a lot more than had I not taken up running! The objective is to live a happy, healthy, long life. For that I'm prepared to pay for nice shoes. There's an old Irish saying:

"Always buy the best mattress and the best shoes you can afford."

There's no need to spend silly money of the really high end shoes. Go for the reasonably priced ones that (a) feel comfortable like a slipper, (b) have a cushioned, gel sole, and (c) pass the fold test.

Chapter 4 - Training begins

Learning from the mistakes

As I mentioned in the preface, it's said that you spend your first two marathons learning how not to run a marathon. If you're anything like me, you'll also spend your early training learning how not to do training. We all learn from our mistakes. You're going to have a bit of trial and error, and you're going to take that in your stride. Early on in my business career I heard about Brian Tracey. One of his quotes is so good that I now apply that to all setbacks, both in business and in life.

> *Quickly say "that's good" to every setback*
> *and then find out what's good about it!*

Like me, you may also be familiar with the age old saying "running a marathon is not like running a sprint". You can (for example) wake up one day and decide that you want to sprint 100 metres. You can go out that morning, and you can do precisely that. Find a 100 metre straight line and run along it. You may not do it well, or be particularly fast, but you're probably going to reach the finish line without pain or discomfort. That's probably not going to be the case with a marathon. Without adequate preparation, you're not going to wake up one day and go out and run a marathon.

The way I see it, you need to train. And you have to do that by following a program which suits *you*. There are hundreds of things out there which will tell you "how" and "what" to do. I wish they had also explained "why". Some of them have sort of helped me, but none of them were really in tune with "an overweight forty something fella" who wants to become fit and do a marathon.

Naturally, any guide you read (including this one) is going to be general purpose and is designed to appeal to a wide audience. If you're lucky enough and rich enough to engage a personal trainer you may get something bespoke. I'm not that rich. In my social circles I've met a couple of personal trainers and their approach revolves around whole body fitness, with a focus on floor exercises and on weights. One of them confided in me that he had never run 10k and was probably never going to be able to run a half marathon let alone a full one. You could be lucky and engage a specialist running coach. If not, you might like to borrow some of my strategies and tailor them to suit your needs.

You can also go onto Runners World and look at their "Marathon Training Plans" page, and probably linger for as long as I did . . . about 5 minutes . . . it starts with "complete beginner" which I am not and then "beginner sub 5 hours" which I honestly think is way too ambitious for a fat middle aged bloke! I don't mean to single out Runners World, as there are lots of other resources like theirs. However, click through to their simplest beginner plan and it shows you an intense 16 week program with four or five runs every week. I don't have the time to do that amount of running, and anyway, I was planning to train over two years not over 16 weeks. The assumption seems to be that you're starting as some kind of ambitious semi professional, rather than the average bloke in the street who wants to be slimmer and fitter. I also get the feeling that these guides are written for people in their twenties and thirties.

I would have to be my own coach.

Turning business coaching into running coaching

So I borrowed a couple of concepts which I use when I work. The first is the old adage:
> *"Failing to plan equals planning to fail."*

Which leads nicely to Peter Drucker's advice to repeatedly "plan, do, review", and his quote "implementation is everything".

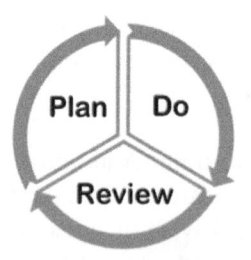

There are two questions which can help any business towards success:

1. If there's one thing you should be doing, but you're not doing, what is that one thing?

2. And, what's stopping you?

You start by addressing whatever is "stopping" you.

Applying the theory

So not only have I become a novice runner, I have also become my own novice running coach. And by giving myself a taste of my own medicine I am now confronted with the awkward questions that I tend to ask others.

Do you know what should be happening and what is actually happening? How do you know? Where's it written down? What metrics have been logged? What changes are you been implementing in order to make things better? Your log will tell you.

I've had a rudimentary exercise log since mid 2005. It became a serious log on 28 Mar 2011 when I put it down on a spreadsheet, and it became more serious still when I added a few more columns and switched from miles to kilometres on 25 Jun 2012. I can only give you these precise dates, because I can look back at my log and I can see what I did and when. I can also see my weight. It peaked on 3 May 2011 giving me a BMI of 30.77 which is just over the threshold and into "obese".

What should be happening is that my weight should be steadily reducing, and I should be in good enough shape to cover 42.195k in less than 6 hours. The cut off time for most official marathons is normally 6 hours. London allows 8 and there are a few others which set a time in the range from 5 hours to 7 hours.

If you're too slow, then you will be compulsorily retired from a race, put on the sweeper bus, and taken to the finish. My task was to accustom my body to longer and longer runs, and to work on endurance. I knew that gradually conditioning my muscles to suit the task was going to be a key ingredient in my success.

I knew what should be happening. Lose weight and cover 42.195k in less than 6 hours. Thanks to a log, a digital watch with a stopwatch, and a set of bathroom scales, I could see what was actually happening.

Plan Do Review

Now it was time to map out a plan. I have, in effect, curated my own self-engineered marathon training policy. I'm suggesting that you do the same. By all means use bits from here and bits from other people, but adjust all the resources you find to suit *your* needs. There is nobody else like you! You are the best qualified person to be you, and you are going to get along fine being your own coach.

In Chapter One I asked you to write down a few things. You might want to take a look at those notes now and ask yourself how you're going to achieve all that? I'm in favour of setting easy targets . . . and hitting them! It took me several years before I committed to completing a marathon. And I decided that I would take my time, I'd train over approximately two years and then I'd do a marathon when I was 50 years old. That would surely be a memory to cherish?

When I embarked on this mad cap plan, I also thought that there would only ever be one marathon!

Couch to 5k

There's a well known system called "Couch to 5k" which is designed to introduce complete beginners to running, without all the pressure and all the stress. Fortunately, I had a head start on all of that. I've always had a fair amount of truly basic running experience.

This book assumes that you're not a beginner, and that you're comfortable covering 5k, whether you can walk it or can run it. I know young healthy people who would rather take the bus than walk two bus stops. Where I live in central London, two bus stops means anything from 300 to 900 metres.

If you need help with "Couch to 5k" then a good place to start is the NHS website. Runners World also has useful material on their website if you look specifically at the "Couch to 5k" category. However, if you already have some basic experience, as I have, or if you've already done the "Couch to 5k" programme, then you're not a complete beginner any more, you're a novice, and that's where the marathon training really starts.

The Gym

I had joined the gym principally to lose some weight, not because I wanted to take up running. Had I not seen the advert for local 10k races in 2005 and 2006, my life would have been quite different. I'm happy with the way things worked out, starting nice and slow, and it was all gentle, low pressure stuff for years and years.

However, the expense of my new found running hobby was mounting up and that wasn't what I had expected. After buying my first pair of "expensive" running shoes, and lots of cheap cushioned socks, I took a moment to take stock.

I was paying for gym membership at a gym where I no longer wanted to run on a treadmill, and it was a gym which had a short 20m swimming pool to boot, not a proper 25m one. The gym had a coach who had been a bit late telling me about running shoes, and I was attending sessions of mixed ability runners all aspiring to complete a 10k race, but all with different running speeds. I needed to get out on the road at a time of my own choosing, and run at a pace which was right for me, not at an average pace for a group. The coach handled mixed ability runners by allowing the slower runners to continue forward in a straight line and periodically instructing the faster ones to turn, run back to where they had just come from, for a distance of two or three lampposts, turn 180°, and then catch up with the slow runners again. In theory that sounds like a helpful mechanism. If nothing else, the concept of measuring distance according to lampposts (or telegraph poles) became cemented in my mind.

What actually happened with that particular group (because I was neither fast nor slow) was that I would turn 180°, run as far as one prior lamppost, abruptly turn 180° again, and then catch up. Mentally that didn't excite me, in fact I hated covering the same ground twice. Later in my running career I made a vow to minimise covering the same ground twice. My ideal race is a single large loop, always covering new ground. Doing a clear "out and back" on the same set of roads is OK, as long as there is a loop at the midpoint - no abrupt 180° turns. Many of my training routes from home are "out and back". They all involve a loop at the midpoint, even if that's just a 60 metre loop circling The Founders Arms on the South Bank of the Thames. The nicest midpoint loop I have is the obvious and natural 2.82k circuit within Battersea Park.

I began to realise that road running is a solitary pursuit, and I preferred being a solo runner. I also prefer to run in the mornings, before having breakfast, and I do not like running during the evenings to suit the gym staff. Evening sessions had too much impact on my normal work and eat and family life routines.

On and off since my twenties, I've had access to four different gyms, and I've never felt that I was getting value from any of them. My gym was always some distance from home and it was usually dominated by fitness fanatics.

Maybe they weren't fanatics, but there was some odd dialogue and some macho behaviour. No matter how well intentioned the comments and the behaviour were (though I suspect some of it wasn't) I found the unwelcome coaching from intimidating men (always men) quite irritating.

On the other hand, my nearest local road was just outside my front door and the joggers I saw were "normal" people. So I decided that in future, my training would start from my front door. The gym membership in 2005 was cancelled as soon as the 3 month promotional price ended.

The Road

Typically I would be out running at about 6am, in my nice new shoes, and all my other bog standard running kit.

Best of all, I was now my own coach, and it was up to *me* to tell *me* how *me* had been doing, and what *me* was going to do next!

A Plan

From what I had read, a marathon is tough, so my plan listed targets for successive Sunday morning runs. Owing to time constraints and my day job I would do short runs on some weekdays, and I would dedicate Sunday mornings to my main run. Typically, but with lots of exceptions, a distance of (say) 10k would be marked up for all the Sundays "this month", and then that would be increased to (say) 12k for all the Sundays "next month".

I trained hard, on roads and paths that I knew, sometimes having Victoria Park in Hackney at one end, and sometimes having Battersea Park at the other, and always having a lot of the "banks of the River Thames" inbetween. That involved crossing various bridges (and regularly negotiating concrete steps) on routes of various distances. Running alongside the river minimises the number of major road junctions you have to negotiate. That's why you see so many people running along The South Bank. If I hadn't known London well before, I certainly know it well now! I also know every single step on the massive staircases at each end of Waterloo Bridge and Southwark Bridge!

Periodically, my plan called for me to enter a formal race. By having a 10k or two in my diary (and later a half marathon) I told myself that I would be more likely to stick to my plan. My spreadsheet had a historic log on Sheet 1. Sheet 2 then became the forward plan, setting out what I was going to do and when. Target setting was limited to "intended distance". I wasn't really concerned about speed, but I did add a few formulae to calculate what my speed was, and then covert that to pace.

For years I had the "speed" mindset not the "pace" mindset. I could relate to 10kmh (which was my ambition, but took some time to achieve) and I found it very hard to identify with the expression "6 minute kilometres". The more I did official races, the easier it became, and it was only when I moved to Geneva in 2016 that I fully grasped the concept of pace. Having waypoints set out in kilometres and not miles was instrumental in that. In major races I fail to understand why the UK will not provide waypoints in both kilometres and miles. How many international runners enter these events? Like me, how many of them train in kilometres? In the UK 5k and 10k races are common. It's time for longer races to use kilometres as well.

My Log

Every time I went for a run, I would come back, sit at my computer, and add some details to the log. Date, time, distance and duration. I soon added a "notes" column where I could record a short narrative like "OK, but too hot, some minor walking". It wasn't exactly a diary, but it was enough to help with "plan, do, review". I soon formed the habit of checking the log before each run, reviewing the last two or three entries, and setting little goals for "today". If I walked a bit last time, then I wasn't going to allow myself to walk this time. I could jog as slowly as anybody could possibly jog, but not permit myself a walking pace.

The log became a fundamental part of my routine. If I was supposed to be out on the road at 6.00am, and I was habitually noting the departure time as 6.20am then I had to do something about motivating myself. Generally I get up at 5.00am, have some tea and read the papers (the online papers). Then I prepare my kit, do my stretches in the kitchen, and get out the door at about 6.00am. The difficulty is when there is too much newsworthy news in the morning!

The log was a valuable, positive, self reinforcing feedback loop. My endurance improved, my weight came down, and my speed and distance went up. The log has continued to be a fundamental part of my training. You can see an example at Appendix 2.

I recommend that you maintain a log. In my case, it's designed in part to incentivise me, to show where I want be performance wise, in terms of distance, speed and weight. It's also an invaluable historical record which helps me make decisions about current and future plans. My log shows a hiatus on two occasions, and getting back on the wagon was made a lot easier by seeing "how did I do it last time". Above all, the purpose of my log is to ensure that my younger self helps my older self. I wouldn't have attempted a third marathon at age 61 if my younger self had not conscientiously documented the journey from when I was 43 years old.

Every tool in my armoury has been employed to make this happen. Once again, my business coaching experience helps with this self-engineered running coaching. Let me give you John Oxley's quote:

> *"Anyone who has managed key performance indicators will tell you, if there is no target for something, the target is zero."*

Your Log

Prepare a log. It makes the chances of success so much better. Base yours on the example at Appendix 2 if you want to. Add and remove bits to suit your needs. Use the metric system, kilometres and kilograms, because that's the norm in the running community. Use it as a key tool in your "plan, do, review" system.

Your older self will be really grateful that your younger self started doing this from today.

Chapter 5 - Techniques, Stretches and Exercises

Health is Threat Management

Doing adequate preparation, before you go out and run, is vital. The right techniques, stretches and exercises will make you more resilient, and will reduce the risk of injury. Don't overdo it, and definitely don't underdo it. Practice makes perfect, and your physical health and mental health will both benefit from taking the time to get this right. Prevention is better than cure. Prevent injuries!

Amongst all of the magnificent and thought provoking books I've read, Georges Canguilhem's *Le Normal et le Pathologique* stands out as a beacon of common sense. The book is actually his PhD thesis, written between 1942 and 1943, when he was working covertly with the French Resistance. It wasn't published (in French) until 1966, and it wasn't published in English until 1989.

Canguilhem was a practising physician, even before he gained his doctorate. His studies at Strasbourg University led him to examine chronicles of medicine, health, psychology and pathology from the mid 1500's to the mid 1900's. His thesis has an emphasis on "the history of ailments" and it was derived from 193 other books and papers, the earliest of which was published in 1780. He's good at explaining "why".

Descartes, another Frenchman, was born at the end of the 1500's. He's best known as a mathematician and a philosopher, yet he also had a great interest in health. In *A Discourse on the Method* he hoped that his "method" would allow him to make progress in medicine:

"as the restoration and maintenance of health and the prevention of the effects of ageing seem to have a place among the highest goods of life"

What Canguilhem is keen to emphasise is that customary definitions of "health" are inadequate, citing the typical definition that "health is the absence of injury, disease, or infirmity". Canguilhem disliked the "absence" definition. He didn't want to know *what health is not*, he wanted to know *what health is*. In 1943 he proposed his own definition.

"Health is threat management, and the ability to adapt to one's environment."

As marathon runners what we're interest in improving our flexibility, our performance and our comfort zone. That means that we need be sceptical of big business selling us goodies which all claim to enhance our health and fitness. To Canguilhem's way of thinking, those who cannot adapt to modern lifestyles, and those who cannot manage the threat from modern foods, may have health issues. Good "threat management" can prevent problems.

In simple terms, it means doing all the things that your mother told you to, or your grandmother. Eat your greens, brush your teeth, and eleventy billion other bits of advice! In my opinion, it also means that you should be suspicious of modern marketing. Eat wisely and exercise wisely. Commercial concerns are not promoting *this product* for your benefit, they're doing it to make profits.

Adam Smith (On the Wealth of Nations, 1776):

> *"It is not from the benevolence of the butcher, the brewer, or the baker, that we can expect our dinner, but from their regard to their own interest."*

My own techniques, stretches and exercises require no specialist equipment at all, this will cost you nothing, and it can be done almost anywhere. My preferred space is my ordinary domestic kitchen in my ordinary domestic home.

My Personal Take

I am wholly unqualified to give you professional advice on stretches and exercises. Seek it out if you wish. Read the caveat at the front of this book again. I'm sharing my facts about my routine. I'm not giving advice.

The purists are probably going to have a go at me, because some of them will disagree with my stretches and exercises routine. It's my routine, my stretches and my exercises, they can advocate what they like, and they can do what they like. You should work out what fits into your own stretches and exercises routine and then you should do whatever you like. That will be better than a lot of people who just sit on the couch and do zero exercise.

Doing your own routine, the way you like it, the way that's in tune with your body, and the way that makes you feel good, is going to have a helpful effect on your physical health Yeo (2021). More than that, it will have a tremendously beneficial effect on your mental health Rosling (2019).

Giles Yeo is a doctor of genetics at Cambridge University. Dr Hans Rosling was a practising physician in his native Sweden. They are both good at explaining "why".

I know what works for me, and I'm sharing it with you, not because I recommend that you adopt my exact routine. I just want my routine to inspire you to go away and figure out what your routine looks like. Select some, all or none of mine. Follow my precise detail if you like, or make up your own precise way of doing it. There are also plenty of other exercises you could try. I'm not able to tell you anything, other than some facts about what I do.

Rule 1

If you don't have time to do your stretches and exercises routine before you run, then you don't have time to run. Shelve it. Wait for another time. You have to prepare your muscles for the task ahead.

I'm guessing you're an adult. You can ignore this and do your own thing. Don't say I didn't warn you!

> *Ethiopian proverb: "Give advice; if people don't listen, let adversity teach them."*

There are no more rules! Make up your own extra rules if you want to.

Self Care

I think of my muscles as a sort of spring like mechanism. If I stretch them, I do so gradually, reaching a point where I still feel in control, sufficiently stressed but not in pain, and I hold it. Like the careful handling of a spring, I release the tension in my muscles slowly. No instantaneous "let go, thank goodness that's all over".

If you release a tensioned spring it can jump unexpectedly. I don't want sudden shocks to my muscles, so as each of my stretches ends I take a few seconds to progressively relax the muscle.

When I was younger I would sometimes go out for a run without first doing my stretches. I sometimes regretted that. With age comes wisdom. Nowadays, I never fail do the stretches first.

I went to proper yoga classes only twice. The less said about that the better. However, I have picked up on some bits of yoga from books and from newspapers, and I have checked the web (YouTube in particular) to try and figure out what on earth some of them are talking about!

Some other bits of dialogue below originate from my mate Tony. Tony and I were at school together. We both left school in 1980 and he went off to join the Royal Air Force. I met him regularly in the years that followed, and he shared news of everything. Especially the physical training. It *was not* quite British Military Fitness (which is a private business founded in 1999) but it *was* the RAF way of doing things. Tony taught me about some of the routines, and (anecdotally) explained that the RAF is a bit less severe than the British Army. Although it was a lot tougher than the PE lessons we had at school!

The 400m track

Tony was keen to get me down to the 400m track at our old school, so that he could show off his improved fitness. During my final year at school I had been chosen by my House to do the 1600m race at sports day. I think I was the only available candidate, and I duly came last. I was a swimmer, occasionally I would win swimming races. I didn't like running!

Anyway, the 400m track at school was open to everyone. You could simply turn up, out of hours, and run around the school fields to your heart's content. Tony didn't want to race me over 1600m, he wanted to do it over 2400m! Six laps of the track.

He explained that during RAF basic training he had been required to do this challenge three times, once at the start of the course, once in the middle, and once at the end. The young recruits were all expected to cover 2400m in 10 minutes 30 or less. If they couldn't do it the first time, then they had to improve. They would fail the whole course if they couldn't achieve 10 minutes 30 or better by the third and final time they tackled the challenge. That was the RAF in the early 1980s. It may be different now.

Both Tony and I had cheap Casio digital watches, the one with the stopwatch, the forerunner of the Casio F-91W which I currently have.

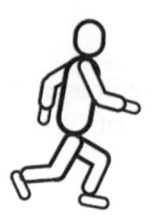

Tony briefed me, and then we set off running together. Gradually a gap developed between us. He finished in less than 10 minutes. I took exactly 10 mins 30 secs measured on both our watches, but only because he shouted at me so much. I have always remembered that day. The promised rematch has never taken place, but I still use this RAF fitness test.

There have been lengthy gaps in my six lap adventures, though periodically I *have* been able to find a local 400m track and put myself to the test. At Versoix just outside Geneva there is easy access to the 400m track at the sports centre.

In London, available to the public in Victoria Park (Hackney), there is an awful 400m track, a mix of mud and cinders. In Regents Park the cinders track is a bit better, but it's narrow and it's only 386.8m long. Regents Park is the one I use nowadays, and I run six laps and a further 80 metres.

I measure the extra 80m in advance, by doing 111 paces at a my normal walking speed, and I set a marker by the side of track. Then I walk back 80m to the start line and set off. When running around the track I've discovered that it's easy to daydream and to forget how many laps I've done. I cannot rely on timing the laps, because I have disciplined myself (over 2400m) to never look at my stopwatch until the end. So to overcome the forgetfulness I wear 6 loose fitting elastic bands on my left wrist, transferring one to my right wrist every time I complete a lap. Problem solved, if I check the number of elastic bands I always know which lap I'm on.

I try to do the 400m track twice a year, every March and every September. During 2024 (a year with irregular training due to injuries) I covered the distance in March in 14 mins 51 secs, and in September in 13 mins 8 secs. A decent uplift for a 61 year old, but the reduced running that year means that I can't read too much into the apparent improvement.

Over the years I have seen my performance on this standard RAF test go up and down. I continue to do it twice a year, because it keeps me up to date with where my fitness stands in general.

Yomping

Having mentioned Tony, I now have to tell you about a military technique called yomping, because it fits nowhere else in this book. Yomping is not part of my stretches and exercises routine, although sometimes it is a part of my running. A little after Tony joined the RAF, the Falklands Conflict broke out. That was in the middle of 1982. The nightly television news would devote a considerable amount of time to coverage of the war. Part way through the conflict, British Forces landed on the islands, and we all learnt a new verb "to yomp".

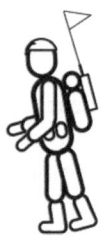

Royal Marine Corporal Peter Robinson

Yomping is Royal Marines slang which describes a long distance forced march carrying full kit. The same thing in the British Army is called "tabbing" meaning "Tactical Advance to Battle".

On television, the Marines' version "yomp" gained the upper hand. It was variously described as running (or jogging) for 100m, then walking (or marching) for the next 100m, and repeating that pattern in order to cover the ground fast. Perhaps that's not a perfect description, but you get the idea.

In the Falklands, a joint operation of Royal Marines and members of the Parachute Regiment (each carrying 36kg of equipment) yomped across rough countryside for 3 consecutive days in order to cover 90k quickly. The original plan had been to use helicopters, but they'd been lost earlier when a Royal Navy ship had been sunk.

Yomping
www.wikipedia.org

The precise explanation (and distances) for "yomping" may vary depending on who you listen to. Elsewhere in this book I use the term "yomping" to describe a pattern of dividing up the ground to be covered, and alternating between running and walking.

When I first used the technique I adopted a pattern of alternating once every 200m. I use roadside lampposts or telegraph poles to regulate my progress. They tend to be spaced out 100m at a time. My 200m pattern is sometimes adjusted to fit different circumstances.

Yomping! Now you know!

Five pre run Stretches

The basic strategy is that I perform each of my five pre run stretches for 20 repetitions, or hold a position for 20 seconds. If it takes a few seconds to get ready, then my 20 second timing does not start until I have the right pose. And I count the seconds in my head, slowly, one and . . . two and . . . three and . . .

Occasionally I check my own timing against the clock in the kitchen. My counting to 20 can sometimes last as long as 30 seconds.

1. The Windmill

Before working my leg muscles, I like to limber up with some arm exercises. And, before starting the windmill, I lift my arms, shake them about, flex my fingers, and generally promote good circulation from my finger tips to my shoulder blades.

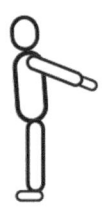

Alternating between each arm and each direction, the right arm starts at the upper most vertical and moves forward in a circular motion for 20 repetitions. Then the left arm. Next the right arm starts at the lower most vertical and moves forward again. Followed by the left one. This way, each arm (and shoulder) is subjected to the fullest possible articulation.

2. Tadasana Gomukhasana

I first tried (and first succeeded in) gripping my hands behind my back during PE lessons at school. That was many, many years before a yoga aficionado introduced me to the expression *tadasana gomukhasana*. It starts with the word *tadasana,* to mean this pose is done whilst *standing* up.

I also massage my shoulders a little before attempting this stretch.

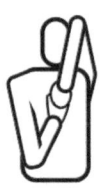

If you can't manage to interlock your fingers don't worry. Can you get your finger tips to touch? The point is to stretch your muscles, and not to be a perfectionist. If your finger tips still refuse to meet, then use a tea towel or a short length of rope. Grip that in both hands, and then pull in order to bring one hand closer to the other. You're looking for gradual improvement, not miracles.

Over time, my performance on this exercise has become better. If you're carrying excess weight this stretch in harder. After I lost a measurable amount of weight (fat deposits around the shoulders) this became much, much easier.

When I first began using this stretch, I found that standing in an open doorway helped. The preparation involved both hands approaching the middle of the back from below, with one hand pushing the other upwards so that it could lie flat between the shoulder blades. An extra push can be obtained by gently forcing your lower elbow against the door frame, giving you just enough help to keep the lower hand in place while you get the upper hand into the correct position.

My target is a good quality "monkey grip" where all the fingers interlock. The more I practice this, the easier it becomes.

3. Calf Muscles

This was a favourite exercise of the sadists I had met (otherwise known as gym instructors). Whilst I was conscientiously making a really good effort to stretch my calf muscle, and to not go to excess, they would persistently and relentlessly demand "more, more".

It's my body and I listen to my body. If I pull a muscle it's me that suffers. In my head I was constantly thinking "it's really taught already - I'm doing as much as I can you absolute muppet - you have no idea how hard I'm trying in order to get to the optimal performance in this stretch".

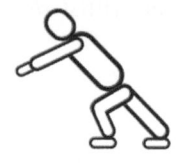

My diplomatic skills won through, and I never actually vocalised my thoughts. If you were coaching me in 2005 then you know who you are, and you played a major role in my decision to give up membership of the gym.

There are multiple ways that you can strike a pose like this. There are also completely different ways to stretch a calf muscle. Sometimes I see runners limbering up for a race by standing upright, raising one leg to the horizontal, resting the heel on a fence, or on the back of a bench, and then gripping the toes with both hands, pulling the end of the foot towards the body whilst keeping the leg perfectly straight. The key is to push the heel away from you, and then bring your toes towards your knee.

The diagram above shows what I look like in my kitchen at home, resting my hands on a work surface. I have never succeeded in pushing the kitchen unit through the wall and into my neighbour's flat, but I am able to stretch the calf muscles effectively. If I'm limbering up near the start of a race, I strike a similar pose by using a big, hefty tree for support.

4. Quadriceps

The point of this exercise is to stretch the front portion of your quadriceps which sit between the knee to the groin. In a perfect world you can get the heel of your foot to touch the buttock.

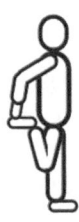

With this position there *is* a temptation to try and achieve two strikes at glory, killing two birds with one stone so to speak. However, the "standing on one leg" test is a separate and unrelated exercise to quads. The quadriceps stretch is there to stretch the quadriceps.

As you get older you may come across the "one legged balance" test. There's one test with your eyes open, and one with your eyes closed. Many illustrations (like the one on the New Scientist website) give you a ridiculous yoga pose to mimic when doing that. The correct pose involves lifting one foot a little, and using the toes of that foot to "wrap" it around the calf of the other leg, just above the ankle. There's a photo on my blog:

Balance Test
www.dontreadmyblog.com

For this quads stretch I invariably go back to the same door frame I mentioned earlier, and I steady myself with one hand resting against the woodwork. Then I concentrate on the correct pose, count to twenty, and actually stretch the quadriceps.

5. Hamstrings

On page 46 I mentioned that I hold each stretch for 20 seconds.

Originally when "touching your toes" I would be using a lot of that 20 seconds just to achieve the correct position. It can take me between 7 and 14 seconds to fully reach down whilst still keep my legs straight. It was this particular stretch that made me refocus on attention to detail. Now, no matter how long it takes for me to get into the right position, I get into the right position first, and then I start counting, and hold it for a further 20 seconds.

The objective is to stretch the hamstring muscles, not to actually touch your toes. You don't have to keep your legs perfectly and rigidly vertical (though that's desirable), you simply need to keep them straight enough to be in character with your normal standing position. The question you have to ask yourself is did you really *stretch those hamstring* muscles? The *biceps femoris*?

Reach down as far as you can. I've seen one exceptional performance from one exceptional person. If you're Mr Bendy Yoga Man try doing this stretch and laying the palms of your hands flat on the floor!

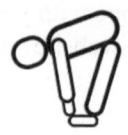

Over time, my own performance on this stretch has improved. Once again, it improved the most after a concerted few months when I had lost a good measure of fat.

Don't overdo it! My philosophy has always been simple . . . I am competing with my younger self . . . I'm not aiming for artistic perfection as if I was some kind of Olympic gymnast or a ballerina!

Two Additional Exercises

Strictly speaking, these extra two exercises are not directly related to running, so they don't have to be performed just before I head out for a run. However, they do feature as part of my weekly fitness regime, and I tend to do sit ups and press ups on the days when I'm not running. My regular routine is to exercise in the early mornings, except on a Saturday, when I have one day off from exercise.

My running timetable includes Tuesdays and Thursdays for a short run before work, and I do my longer runs on Sundays. That means that sit ups and press ups are for Mondays, Wednesdays and Fridays. I like routines, and I like to stick to routines!

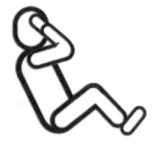

And although they are unconnected with running, these exercises are logged on the same spreadsheet. One fitness record. That way, when I look back at my performance I can see everything in one place showing me how I've improved.

The sit ups are done the way I was taught, as a school kid, in the 1970s. Some argue that I'm doing them wrong. I don't care! I just go and do them wrongly, and it improves my stomach muscles and the overall tone of my torso.

Typically, I do this at home in the kitchen, or in the office at my desk. My toes are hooked under the lip of a kitchen unit, or under the drawer pedestal of my desk. If you can't find somewhere to anchor your feet, then a companion can be persuaded to hold your feet down at the ankles. You can do sit ups without being anchored, I just prefer to keep my feet still.

Adopting the pose shown in the illustration, my fists are lightly clenched, with fingers placed against the temples, and thumbs nearest the ears. Without excessive movement of the arms or legs, my head, neck and torso do the hard work, with the greatest demand being placed on stomach muscles. There is no compulsion to do these quickly, nor to do 20 in a row without stopping. The important thing is to work the stomach muscles and improve them. The sit up starts with the back of my head resting on the floor, the midpoint is when my elbows touch my knees, and the end is when the back of my head reaches the floor again.

The final sit up is not finished until I return my head to the floor, nice and slowly, giving the stomach muscles one final, demanding task.

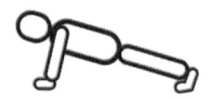

With press ups it's usually 20 at a time. What's important to me is "the form". Body straight, legs parallel, fingers not splayed, hands parallel and pointing forwards, in line with the shoulders. The hands are sufficiently far apart so that at the raised point, the elbows form a nice 90° angle. As the body moves lower I go far enough for the tip of my nose to briefly touch the floor, and then I rise again, no resting between individual press ups, and no torso on the floor.

To me, "the form" means getting it to look right and feel right, and getting the maximum benefit from the exercise. It's not about doing it quickly or getting in more reps in order to impress somebody else. I'm doing it for *me*, and I want be satisfied with *my* health and fitness.

In Chapter 8 you will see the story of the Black Belt in Karate who concentrates on "the form". I am not obsessive about "the form", but I support the general idea. I am always conscious of doing disciplined movement, not particularly with my running style, but especially with my sit ups and press ups. Getting "the form" *correct* is the objective. I am not trying to get "the form" *perfect*, nor should you.

Pain

If it hurts, stop.

That's easier said than done! If you know exactly where the pain is, then it's easy to stop the one thing that causes that one pain. The alternative is to stop everything and get some proper advice. That's also easier said than done!

At stretches 1 and 2 above I described how I routinely do The Windmill and Tadasana Gomukhasana before each training run. One day, as this case study explains, things didn't go to plan.

> **The Weird Shoulder Pain**
>
> During a 10k run on Sunday 15 Jul 2012 I had a weird pain in my left shoulder. I naturally blamed my excessive enthusiasm with that morning's stretches.
>
> I finished the run as normal, and decided to take it easy for a while so that I could let the shoulder muscle recover. The problem was that I had pain in more than one place. And if you have multiple pain points you only really notice the one that shouts loudest. I went to see my GP three times.
>
> Then, one morning at 5.00am I woke in such pain that I went to A&E at my local hospital (where I waited for 3 hours). Two weeks after that it was so bad that I went to A&E again, mid afternoon, and I was seen more quickly. None of the professionals identified what the issue was. It took me about six weeks of pain and personal research for me to self diagnose RSI.
>
> Repetitive Strain Injury
> www.dontreadmyblog.com
>
> Use the QR code to read the whole story on my blog. It was absolutely nothing to do with my running or stretching routines! And it was simply an unfortunate coincidence that I first noticed the pain during an early morning run.

Having once been so overweight that I was technically obese, my strategy now is to minimise risk. Don't overdo it, and don't underdo it. The techniques, stretches and exercises I've adopted are all designed to help me stay healthy, and to live up to what Canguilhem said.

"Health is threat management, and the ability to adapt to one's environment."

That applies to my running, to my diet, and to the arrangement of furniture and equipment in my home and my office. To everything! It's up to you to find the right system for you. Just remember, if you don't have time to do your stretches before you run, then you don't have time to run.

Chapter 6 - Race Preparation

Building a Plan

Failing to plan equals planning to fail.

When the astronauts first went to the moon, they had one flight plan, and one million in flight adjustments, so the saying goes. Preparing for a first marathon has a lot in common with that. Having a plan is important. Being prepared to adjust that plan, while it's actually in progress, is even more valuable.

Chapter 4 was about adopting running as a pastime. Chapter 6 is about making a commitment and a plan to complete a marathon. Both of these chapters stress the importance of planning. In my case, getting serious about running took me years. Six years, from 2005 to 2011. Throughout that time there was always a vague, whimsical notion that I might one day do a marathon.

My log shows that I took the plunge on 29 May 2012. I committed to the genuine prospect of running a marathon. The London marathon (22 Apr 2012) had taken place recently. The city was awash with and preparations for the 2012 Olympics. And "sport" was at the forefront of everybody's mind. What I needed was a robust plan, with a set of incremental goals, so that I could implement it with a minimal risk of failure.

Begin With the End in Mind

Stephen Covey tells us what to do in his book *The 7 Habits of Highly Effective People*. Begin with the end in mind. I needed to choose a marathon, and I knew from the start that it was *not* going to be London, because I didn't want all the fuss and fanfare. Going anywhere on public transport during major events is tough, let alone joining a mass start of 50,000 people in Greenwich Park. As a first timer I was worried about finding my comfort zone in a race of that size.

April 2013 looked like a good option. That would give me nearly a year to prepare, and the event would be roughly six months after my 50th birthday. Now all I needed was a location. Not too far from home, and nothing with an excess of razzamatazz. Brighton looked right! It was scheduled for 14 Apr 2013.

The Brighton Marathon was inaugurated in 2010, so it would be the fourth time the event was staged. The race had around 8,000 runners in each of the its first two years, and the one that had just passed in 2012 had amassed a field 12,000 runners. Big enough to be serious, yet small enough not to intimidate me. I know Brighton a bit. In spite of a few tiny hills, it's a relatively flat place, it's a one hour train ride from London, and I could easily get there and back on the same day. And most importantly, I could be on an early train and in Brighton in plenty of time for the start. Brighton had a six hour cut off, and that was my big challenge. I really wanted to finish, and my target was "finish before you get picked up by the sweeper bus".

On 11 Jun 2012, two weeks after promising myself that I would actually do a marathon, I duly paid £67.50 and entered the 14 Apr 2013 Brighton Marathon. There was no turning back now, that was a hefty fee, so I wanted to be sure I would get my money's worth.

Breaking it Down

With roughly one year to prepare, my plan quickly evolved around three key factors. I was making this up as I went along. I hadn't been happy with advice from the gym, nor was I happy with the online resources which seemed to focus on people much younger than me. People who might have only 16 weeks to get ready and who wanted to do the distance in around 4 hours.

Hence, I was building my own "three factor" plan for me, from scratch:

- Incremental - target distances
- Stamina - being physically prepared
- Strategy - being mentally prepared

These factors were all equally important to me, and I knew that my plan had to be broken down into stages. Gradually increasing my distance so that I could cover the course. And to be able to do that at a respectable pace so that 50 year old me could finish a marathon in less than 6 hours. You've heard the expression "it's a marathon, not a sprint". Well, you need to keep that in mind as you prepare for your first marathon.

Back in 2006 when I elected to do my first 10k race, that distance alone had seemed like a marathon task to me! I was certain that I could do it, because other people can do it, but I simply had no idea how much effort would be needed. I completed one official 10k race in 2006, two in 2007, and a number of others over the years. I also routinely ran 10k as part of my personal training plan.

Persuaded by a friend to help out with a charity, I did my first half marathon in 2007 and wished I hadn't. I waited a long time before I tackled another half marathon (early 2013) and that was only because my marathon plan said that I had to do one! The 2007 race was the only time that I paid a bit more to contribute to charity. Generally I pay the entry fee and I do not get involved in charity fund raising. I already, routinely, support my favourite charities.

I can't tell you where I picked up the comment "if you can do three quarter distance in training, then you can do the full distance on the day", but it stuck with me in those early days. And not knowing any better, I went along with the myth of three quarter distance. It gets a mention on the Sri Chinmoy and the Run & Become websites, and they both attribute it to some unspecified "classic marathon training" documentation. Anyway, I foolishly believed it, and I foolishly rounded down three quarters of a marathon (from 31.65k) down to 30k.

I was planning to increment my distances so that by the Sunday before the Brighton Marathon I would be able to cover 30k in about 4 hrs 15 mins.

It might have been better if I had adopted the "full distance" strategy which I did before my first 10k race in 2006. In short, I did the full distance on a training run before doing the race itself. Back then I had done lots of 5k and 6k runs in training. Six weeks before race day I did a three quarter distance run in 51 minutes. Three weeks before race day I completed a full 10k training run in 73 minutes. Those were the timings without the luxury of closed roads.

On race day I had an uninterrupted journey around the 10k route. My finish time was 64 mins 25 secs. Not especially impressive in the grand scheme of things, yet for me it was a major achievement back in 2006.

If you have a marathon lined up imminently, then you need a pen and paper now, and you need to write this down. Put a date in the top corner. You'll really appreciate having dated documentation when you're looking back at this stuff later. Map out a rough plan now, it'll change over time, but just write down now what you think your incremental plan should look like from now to the big day.

What distances are you going to do? And when? And what would be a realistic time for you? We're talking about SMART goals. If you've not see that before have a quick look at Wikipedia. I've found the SMART goals concept particularly helpful in my work and in my private life.

SMART goals
www.wikipedia.org

Paul's Timeline

The timeline I drafted was deliberately lop sided, making my training pattern more intense the nearer it was to marathon day. The twofold approach was to progress:

- slowly from 10 to 21.097k
- rapidly from 21.097 to 30k

The reason for the imbalance is that I didn't want to spend lots of time doing longer distances. A few weeks for the second phase was (I foolishly believed) going to be enough. I still had to balance work and family life with my newfound determination to pursue my ambition.

I read about marathon training again, about rest days, about carb loading, and once again I was disappointed to find that nobody was offering advice for middle aged men with excess fat, and a poor track record.

In addition to the running, I also started walking to work on some days, and usually taking the Tube home. Sometimes I would walk the journey in both directions. In those days the journey from home to office was 8k. I ran it a few times. I even worked out a 10k route, crossing the River Thames to the South Bank and crossing back again. I ran that a few times, but mainly I walked it, doing the journey regularly over the summer of 2012.

Timeline 10 to 21.097k

In order to improve my stamina, my longer runs on Sundays went up gradually from 10k to 12, then 14, then 16, and so on. The precise distances were a little different, because (a) I was selecting routes which naturally fitted the roads in my neighbourhood, and (b) I was still measuring things in miles in the early days. My 16k route was actually recorded in my log as 10.27 miles (or 16.45k) with Albert Bridge at one end and the Millenium Bridge at the other.

Much later, I switched to using kilometres for everything. I wish I had done that from the start. If you're starting now, select one or other and stick to it. It makes comparing your notes so much easier!

All of those modest runs passed off without a problem, and whilst I was slow, I could do distances up to 16k, and I could hit my target times.

I also wanted to be ready mentally, and had decided that entering more official races was going to help me develop the right mindset.

In the later part of 2012 I had booked myself onto a 10k race in Deal, Kent, and another in Victoria Park, Hackney. The one on the coast in Deal had an uncharacteristically hilly inland route. I wasn't used to hills and I hadn't trained for them. The race took me 66 mins 05 secs. The Victoria Park 10k was the first one I ever did which involved multiple laps. Three and a half laps of the park. All flat, so I had a good time, 59 mins 32 secs. But it was dull, it lacked atmosphere and it was populated by runners and marshals who demonstrated absolutely no camaraderie whatsoever, with anybody!

In contrast to the handful of other races I had done that had shocked me, and I resolved not to do that event ever again. I had tried to start conversations before and after the Victoria Park 10k, but gained the feeling that "this is not how things are done here".

The Bishops Park, Fulham event was similar. I wasn't on form for a 10k that day and I took a ridiculously long 71 mins 45 to cover the course. I was so slow that the marshals were visually perturbed by my tardiness. I know they're all volunteers, but a hint of a smile, and some fleeting encouragement would have been welcome. The races I do outside London are a lot more friendly than the ones in the central boroughs.

With both stamina and mental fitness in mind, I booked a place on the Wokingham Half Marathon for 10 Feb 2013. I was primed and ready to do that distance. Although it rained! Not heavily, but it was proper rain, and it was the first time I had ever run in proper rain. I didn't have suitable wet weather running kit so I improvised. That morning I prepared my T shirt with the bib safety pinned in place, and I selected my lightweight kagool. I also elected to wear my tracksuit trousers. As I drove from London to Wokingham I was vainly hoping for the rain to ease off. It didn't!

On arrival I parked in the designated muddy field, and thought this through again. What exactly should I wear and how? I would need rain protection throughout the run I thought. I decided that rather than push safety pins through my (not quite waterproof) waterproof kagool, I would wear my T shirt over the top of it. And that meant wearing the cheap polyester kagool right next to my skin.

A bag drop was available in large tents in the muddy field next to the muddy car park. I had a change of clothes and shoes with me, all old stuff which I could afford to lose, and all packed into a small, cheap draw string bag. With my tag attached to the bag, I duly left it in the correct place, on a wet muddy coir mat on the wet muddy grass.

As we gathered at the pens for the start, I noticed that the experienced runners were wearing black bin bags. Suitably modified, one bin bag served as a temporary rain proof jacket, and another as a set of leggings. Then, momentarily before the race started, these were cast off to one side for the volunteers to tidy up. I made a mental note to use this strategy in future, though I was still unsure if I would cope running in wet weather the way that they do. Wearing just shorts and a short sleeved shirt. Around 90% of the field did that. None of my training had involved proper rain, only the lightest of showers, and it made me think that I needed to deliberately go out and do a training run in the rain. Perhaps the next time I have a rainy morning in London!

It rained on and off throughout the Wokingham Half. Every time there seemed to be a lull in the rain you gained a false sense of security, before the rain promptly resumed. My socks and feet were wet within moments of the start. Once you have wet feet you just have to persevere. To minimise discomfort I spent a lot of the race trying to stick to the centre of the road, using the camber to my advantage, and avoiding the water which gathered at the edges.

In spite of the rain, the marshals were stoically cheerful and I appreciated that greatly. Sign posting was fine, and the water stations were wisely positioned and well resourced. From an organisational point of view this was much better than any of the 10k races I had done in and around London.

I completed the race in 2 hrs 36 mins 6 secs. Had it been dry I could have probably beaten my 2 hour 30 target, but in the circumstances I was very pleased with that time. I finished very much towards the back of the field, so the bag drop was largely empty when I arrived. That meant my bag was obvious and I was especially pleased to see that it hadn't vanished.

With rain still coming down, I performed some minor gymnastics getting changed in the car! I was really grateful to have a full set of dry clothes to wear on the journey home.

Timeline 21.097 to 30k

Still believing in the myth of "if you can do three quarter distance in training, then you can do the full distance on the day" I had allowed myself roughly two months to increase my distance up to 30k.

In increments of roughly 2k I followed my plan. The week after the Wokingham Half I did an easy 22k. Then a 25k run in 3 hrs 5 mins and 38 secs, and another 25k in 3 hrs 0 mins and 16 secs. The next increment was supposed to be a further 5k to get me to 30k. Was 30k going to be enough? That's slightly less than three quarter distance and I was thinking there's still a big gap between that and

42.195k. Would I have the stamina to do a marathon if I didn't train for longer distances?

Instead of rounding down I would round up. And remember, I was logging thing in miles back then. I could do my 10 mile route twice? But I detest covering the same ground twice, so I didn't want to do two laps of that route. I worked out a 20 mile training run covering new ground, taking me around many of my familiar places, and this time taking me into and around Hyde Park as well. It was just over 20 miles, or just short of 33k.

It would soon be time for the Brighton Marathon and I had planned to run my new 33k route on Sunday 31 Mar 2013, just two weeks before the race. But the plan didn't go to plan! Because I had been emailed final joining instructions for the Brighton race.

What they didn't tell me until three weeks before race day was that I had to be in Brighton one day early in order to pick up my race pack in person from the "Marathon Village". Unlike all the other races I had done, they would not post race packs, in any circumstances. I phoned. I had to be there on the Saturday to collect the bib and timing chip. Mr Intransigence was not wavering. Not even if I paid P&P and paid extra for Special Delivery.

That meant that I either had to travel by train on two consecutive days, or I would need a Brighton hotel for the Saturday night! No way! I already had plans for the Saturday 14 Apr 2013. I was distinctly unimpressed at being told the arrangements so late in the day, and I really didn't want to fork out any more money for a second train journey, or for a hotel.

I looked for another marathon at short notice. Paying another entry fee was going to be cheaper than paying for one night in a Brighton Hotel! I phoned the organiser of the Milton Keynes Marathon and my only real question was "will you post me the race pack"? Yes!

Brighton was off, Milton Keynes was on.

On 10 Apr 2013 I paid £45.98 and entered the 6 May 2013 Milton Keynes Marathon. That was the May bank holiday Monday. The event was taking place for only its second time. It was a single circuit, no laps, and it was a small event with around 5,000 entrants.

With a bonus of three extra weeks to train I eased off a little, and I left my new 33k route until 28 Apr 2013, just 8 days before race day. That training run was uneventful, run at a very gentle pace, no massive effort, and I was pleased with the time of 4 hrs 17 mins and 4 secs. Although getting from Battersea Park to

Hyde Park is not a route that I'd recommend for runners, and I've never done it again.

Not only were my training run times up where I wanted them to be, the Milton Keynes Marathon had a 6 hour 30 cut off as opposed to the 6 hour limit for Brighton. Everything was feeling good.

I half know Milton Keynes in the same way that I half know Brighton. I could get there and back by train on the same day, and there were no engineering works interfering with travel on the bank holiday. My year of training had pretty much gone to plan. My weight had come down by several kilos. And I had found a forecasting tool on *www.runnersworld.com*

The forecaster required the details of several recent long runs that I'd done. It used all that data to estimate my likely marathon time. The forecast said 5 hrs 42 mins 14 secs. Fine by me! Better than the regular 6 hour cut off which was what I was conscious of when planning for Brighton. In any case Milton Keynes allowed a more generous 6 hour 30 cut off. I was 50 years old, and I was going to complete my first marathon.

I was ready.

Chapter 7 - Marathon 1 Milton Keynes

Bank Holiday Monday 6 May 2013

By the time I decided that I was actually going to do my first marathon I had lived in the centre of London for about 20 years. I know the place really well, and that's one of the reasons that the London Marathon was not going to be my marathon of choice. I needed less razzamatazz, less pressure, and less attention. My younger brother completed the London Marathon in 2001 and was in no hurry to do another one. He was young in 2001 and his time was a respectable 3 hrs 25 mins.

UK marathons are generally laid out with waypoints in miles. Twenty six of them. The precise half way point is usually marked at 13 and a bit, and they end at exactly 26 miles and 385 yards. However, I did the latter part of my training in kilometres. Almost every runner I know keeps records in kilometres. Your local Park Run on a Saturday is 5 kilometres. Yet the marathon organisers in this country persist is using miles and setting the waypoints in miles. In this chapter, I will use kilometres, referring only to miles when discussing the waypoints which I saw along a 42.195k marathon course.

I've been to Milton Keynes many times, to visit family, to see friends, and (just occasionally) to work at the training facilities at Kents Hill. Milton Keynes is one of those New Towns that were designed in the 1960s, and the car is king. They make a virtue of their cycling provision too, with dedicated cyclepaths which are called Redways. In many places the surface has red tarmac to signify cyclepath or "Redway". And the people who organise the Milton Keynes Marathon make a virtue of these cyclepaths by highlighting that it "involves far less of the invariant grade road running that is typical elsewhere". I hadn't read all of the material on their website before the race, because I had only selected Milton Keynes at the last minute.

I had been expecting to run in Brighton on Sunday 14 Apr 2013. I know my way around Brighton a little better than I know my way around Milton Keynes. They had something in common though, both the Brighton and Milton Keynes Marathons were relatively new fixtures on the calendar, having commenced in 2010 and 2012 respectively.

The Redways in Milton Keynes are awful. I have a Brompton folding bike. Using the Redways I once cycled the recommended route from the railway station to the Kents Hill conference centre. The sign posting is dire, with not a single helpful sign as you emerge from the station to unfold your bike. Unless we're talking about the three or four signs which greet rail users with a big red "no cycling" prohibition.

When you eventually manage to levitate yourself and your prohibited bicycle far enough away from the railway station, over the footpath, and the taxi rank, and the bus station, and a further large expanse of piazza, you might be lucky enough to actually find where the Redway actually starts. I never have. After dozens of visits I still don't know where it starts. I've never worked out how cyclists are supposed to leave and arrive at the station unless they walk the first/last 200m.

At one point during my journey to Kents Hill I was cycling along a Redway, on an S shaped path, which ran through a field of sheep. That meant negotiating gates and cattle grids at each end. The field was perfectly rectangular, and the route takes you diagonally from one corner to another. A perfectly straight line, and some looney has decided that what the cyclists need is an S shaped cyclepath across a field! To get back to the railway station I cycled on the roads!

On the day of the marathon my wife and my 11 year old son came with me. We all cycled from home to Euston station (a route we know well), took the train north, and then cycled the unfamiliar Redways as we made our way to the Dons' Stadium.

Oh dear, these particular Redways are in a bad state! I hadn't been here before. The undergrowth at each side was encroaching severely onto the paths. Cyclists had about two thirds of the original width available. The tarmac surfaces were appalling, pitted, loose, and unloved. In places I imagined that they had been laid down in 1960 and had never been touched since. There were few sign posts for any destination at all. The sign posting for the stadium was predictably awful. Cyclists are clearly at the bottom of the priority list at Milton Keynes Council.

Little did I know that later in the day I would be running considerable distances on these deteriorating Redways. The marathon route also included a few stretches of grass, uneven foot paths, canal paths, gravel tracks (I don't run on gravel), and (unbelievably) two humpback bridges.

It was a course formed as a single loop though. And that was a key factor in choosing this race and not the one in Gravesend, which goes around the 8,500 metre Velo Park multiple times. At some stage after 2013, the arrangement in Milton Keynes changed, and it's now two laps of a smaller course.

The bank holiday weather was fine, there was a fair bit of sunshine, no rain, and the sort of temperatures and cloud cover that I was accustomed to. I had trained for this. Having completed one long 33k run eight days earlier I was certain that I could do the distance.

Based on John Backley's strategy I was in no hurry. My target time was 5 hours 59 or better. Milton Keynes has an unusual 6 hour 30 cut off time. Most marathons stipulate 6 hours. Exceptionally, London allows 8 hours. In Milton Keynes we were warned that that the sweeper bus would collect anyone who was not on target to finish within 6 hours 30. Enforced retirements could be invoked by the marshals at any stage after the half way point, if you were deemed to be so slow that making up the time would be improbable. I knew this a few weeks beforehand. The more generous cut off time was also a factor in my last minute choice of Milton Keynes. I had worked out that that if I had problems running, I could power walk 42.195k within 6 hours 30!

Optimistically, I had calculated that I was on for a time of about 5 hours, and would hopefully finish in less than 5 rather than exceed it. For this race I wore tracksuit trousers, a T shirt, a sweatband, and I was on my second pair of running shoes, the New Balance N2. I also used a bum bag for carrying my phone, lip salve, five £10 notes, and a tiny plastic pouch of water. My wife looked after my keys, jacket and sundry stuff. There were changing facilities (massive, temporary changing facilities) available at The Dons' Stadium, and there was a bag drop.

As I left the stadium to walk the short distance to the start I was met by four Stormtroopers. None of us had seen this before and my son, being a typical Star Wars fan, ensured that we stopped for photos. Most of the runners and the crowds were ahead of us. I was happy to be at the back, I was in no hurry. That ensured that we had the four Stormtroopers all to ourselves. Until one of them pointed out that I had better get a wiggle on as the gun had been fired and the race had started!

When I joined the 5 hour starting pen, the first runners had set off, and we were already shuffling forward. I approached the start line, I waved farewell to my loved ones, and I set off. Slowly! I crossed the start line, my chip presumably registered, because I deliberately placed my foot on the sensors, and I hit the start button on my stopwatch.

There were lots of runners failing to get into their stride, hopping, walking, skipping, shuffling a bit more, looking for a bit of clear road to help them settle into their normal pace. I should have joined the 6 hour starting pen, as a few hundred others had. We were all a bit cramped in the 5 hour group.

After watching the start, my wife and son spent most of the day at the hotel in the stadium complex. Lounge, restaurants, bar, toilets, and plenty of scope for food and drink. I planned to call them at the midpoint of the race, and then later on when I was a couple of miles from the finish.

If there was a waypoint marker at Mile One it had vanished by the time I arrived. That was unsettling, I couldn't check my stopwatch at the right place. I wasn't alone in this, other runners around me were also confused. We were sure that we had passed one mile and we would have to wait another 12 minutes or so to try and clock the next waypoint.

I know that there are official photographers at these big events. Usually at the finish, and maybe at a couple of other significant spots en route. It would be nice to have one of those official photographs, proof that I did it, just in case my first marathon is my last marathon. Before starting I had thought "be prepared" for the official photographers.

But not at 5k I thought!

Without warning, I stumbled across a photographer at about 5k. Obviously an official photographer, he was on the runners' side of the barrier, sat on a low folding stool, pointing a fancy camera at every runner who approached. With barely enough time to move clear of the runner in front of me, I hurriedly offered a thumbs up and a gormless smile. It's the only official photo of me there is, so I ended up buying it.

Somewhere between Mile 5 and Mile 6 I had a shock. What I had not expected was a multi terrain course! And I didn't find out until we all turned left, off the road and onto the grass. What? Grass? Seriously? I had no idea how long this would last. However, my initial fears were short lived after we covered just 50 metres of grass and joined a paved footpath near the main hospital. However, how many more grass stretches was I going to encounter? And what other surprises were in store for me?

Lots!

What I hadn't trained for was taking on water or energy gel at the correct intervals. I was relying on the water stations dotted around the course. The tiny pouch of water in my bum bag was an emergency supply. Two mouthfuls if I was lucky, but it was comforting to know that it was there if all else failed. I was planning to take on water at the official water stations. That's what I had always done before, during 10k races and half marathons.

Anyway, I had never seen energy gel sachets before so foolishly I tried one, at about the 10k mark, together with half a cup of water. That was a bad decision! The liquids sloshing around in my stomach disrupted my rhythm and it took ages to get back into my regular stride. I'm not sure that I ever did!

Somewhere at about 16k the course went through a modern housing estate, on the North East side of the town. There were parking spaces in a neat arrangement in the middle of the houses, and among that was the local radio station. Two cars from the outside broadcast team, and one presenter who was doing his best to interview the runners in two second slots! I slowed down to a walk.

"Hi, what's your name?"
"Proactive Paul."
"And that's Proactive Paul, number 2711, going past us now."

Two words! The shortest radio interview I've ever done!

I was slower than intended. I never recovered my composure after failing to get a time check at the missing Mile One post. I had checked my watch at Mile Two, did some mental arithmetic, and nothing made sense. I had reached Mile Two in 20 minutes when it ought to have been something like 24. Worse than 24 to be honest, because we had spent the first few hundred metres trying not to bump into one another. My pace was clearly slower than normal. So, was the Mile Two post in the wrong place? Other runners concurred, it was all a bit confusing.

My marathon had started badly with the first two waypoints being missing and/or off plot. Then after the stupidity of the gel and water intake at about 10k I gave up even trying to work out where I should be in my mental map of the event. No more mental arithmetic was required. As long as there were quite a few people behind me, I reckoned I was OK.

After the midpoint at 21k I checked my stopwatch and it said 2 hrs 38 mins 52 secs. That was three minutes more than it took me to do the Wokingham Half, and this news was the second good thing that happened to me that day!

The first was the photo opportunity with the Stormtroopers! The second was my time at the mid point.

At the half way stage I was so content that I took a full cup of water, relaxed a little and allowed myself some walking. I phoned my wife to give her an update.

At water stations plenty of the runners slow down, take water, walk a bit, chuck the disposable cup and start running again. I finished the water, and walked for much longer that I should have. I ran again, water sloshing around a bit too much inside me, oops, stop running, start walking again!

I had told myself earlier that no more mental arithmetic was required. Well think again Paul, if you're going to walk like this, you had better start building a new plan right now. Just 21k left to go and you have 3 hours 50 in which to do it. Power walking the remainder of the course is possible, but that wasn't in my plan, and in any case, this gentle stroll you're doing right now is *not* power walking! And for goodness sake, stop gulping down too much water!

Willen Lake is a place I know. The course led us into the park on the north side, near the hospice. It's a park with a lovely tarmac path heading south for a good 1,500m and it was crowded with Bank Holiday visitors. There were tiny kids on small bicycles, babies in buggies, youngsters overdosed on sugar, shouting and running around like lunatics, and there was no segregation for runners. Perhaps it was segregated earlier. There was a line, notionally marked on the tarmac surface, but by the time I arrived it was a free for all.

To the public we few runners were just insignificant tail enders, no matter that we were pretty exhausted. They were totally indifferent. A crazy sort of weave was required to negotiate my way through the people in the park. I didn't want to run on the grass and risk an ankle injury. I seemed to be doing a troubled dance along this 1,500m and that made me even more unhappy. There I was trying to make good progress at my pathetic jogging speed, and there was the great Milton Keynes public out in the park trying to, and perfectly entitled to, have a pleasant bank holiday Monday afternoon.

Who organises a marathon like this I thought? Well, this is only the second time the Milton Keynes event has ever been staged, maybe last year's was worse? As I emerged from the mayhem at Willen Lake I phoned my wife again.

I walked a little, I ran a lot, I walked a little more, and I ran as often as I could. I now had no idea where I was. This is a corner of Milton Keynes that I had never seen before, it has a canal, and there were no barriers, no signs, no segregated space, and the runners were mingling with assorted pedestrians as we progressed along the left hand side of a canal. I say "runners", at that stage there were only three of us in our tiny group, no runners visible ahead, and none visible behind. And the three of us shared the same yomping strategy, walk a little bit, run a significant bit, walk a little bit, and so on.

We were running along a concrete tow path, on the left of the canal, and it was covered in a significant layer of mud and gravel, probably carried along by some of the cyclists whose tyre tracks meandered in and out of the muddy space beside the concrete path. We saw another of today's waypoints, Mile 18, so clearly we were still on the right course. A bit further along, the path connects with a humpback bridge, no signs, and there were footpaths on each side of the canal. What do we do? The three of us agreed "straight on", stick to the left hand side of the canal, if they had wanted us to cross the canal (on a humpback bridge of all things) then they would have sign posted it for us. We continued straight on for another 300m, until a chap on the right hand side started shouting at us, "wrong way"!

Was he a race official? No, just an ordinary bloke in ordinary clothing, but he was adamant "other runners have passed me on this side" he shouted. What would you do? The three of us stopped. Utterly incredulous at this apparent cock up! If it was indeed a cock up. Should we believe this stranger? Should we have crossed that bridge? But there was no sign post! Were we supposed to have crossed an earlier bridge, had we missed an earlier signpost that was actually there? Do we keep going straight in the hope of rejoining the course, or do we double back?

And what if the route *is* on the other side *and* also diverges from the canal before we get to the next bridge? That was the killer question. We also had no idea if and when there would be another bridge.

We doubled back, cursing beneath our breath, but thanking Mr Shouty Man for his advice. He stuck around as we retraced our steps, back 300m, over the humpback bridge, forward 300m again. He was still there and we thanked him again. His entire conduct seemed totally authentic, and we were absolutely satisfied that he had told us the truth.

Mind you, we weren't happy. By doubling back we had just covered 600m more than we had to. As I recall, I was in a worse mood than the other two, they had done marathons before and were trying to offer me encouragement as best they could. I told them that when we reached the next marshal I would have to stop, I was badly fatigued, I wanted to regain my composure, and in any case I needed a break for a minute or two. I didn't explain fully, but I also needed a break to number crunch my revised timing and strategy. Some proper mental arithmetic was well overdue. Besides that, I was going to be walking a lot more, and I wasn't going to be able to match my companions' pace to the end.

We ran a bit further along the canal, the left hand path vanished, and there was just the one tow path on our side of the canal. Mr Shouty Man had been right, we were now on the correct side of the canal. As we progressed we could see another humpback bridge further ahead. Getting closer we could also see that there was a marshal on the other side.

Whether there was a sign post at this latest bridge or not, I don't remember, and it didn't really matter because clearly we had to cross the bridge and go past the marshal. We crossed, my two companions carried on, and I stopped. I resisted the urge to tell a volunteer marshal how upset I was. It wasn't his fault and I didn't have the energy, and anyway, it would have been futile. I simply said "I'm going to stop for a minute, probably two or three minutes, don't worry, I need to get some blood to my head, so I'm going to lie down on this slope with my feet upwards and my head downwards, don't worry. If I don't get up after three minutes, then worry"!

That's exactly what I did, I lay down on a bit of grass beside the path, feet pointing up towards the humpback bridge. I closed my eyes and slowly counted to 180, and then I slowly sat up, sat around for another couple of minutes to do some mental maths, and took into account this extended five minute rest time, the time still available, and the remaining distance. It was a healthy, reassuring mental arithmetic exercise and I was ready. I could do this. I phoned my wife once more, and briefly explained the delay. I had done the numbers, I would finish within 6 hours 30.

By carefully planning to yomp the final 12k, I could beat the sweeper bus. Having left the marshal by the canal I was now pretty much on my own. There were fleeting encounters with other runners, but none matched my pace or strategy, so we'd just nod as each of them overtook me.

Without being forewarned, I now encountered the most sensationally dire bit of the Redways. Roughly 10k of badly maintained, crumbling tarmac set alongside the main roads.

Milton Keynes also has a lot of roundabouts. As you encounter each consecutive junction these Redways go up, down, left and right, and through all sorts of permutations to take you through cycle underpasses, and over cycle bridges. Sometimes they pass through the centre of the roundabouts, and sometimes they take you around them in a massive arc. The ones going through the centres of roundabouts bugged me with the constant repetition of up and down. There may be hardly any natural hills in Milton Keynes, but all of these minor ascents and descents add up. As I said earlier, I do my training largely on the Thames Path in London. I'm not used to ascents and descents, and certainly not 10k of them all strung together, each one a short but tedious combination of a drop and a climb every few hundred metres! And that's on neglected, unloved surfaces that most cyclists wilfully avoid.

Imagine a scene from a *Doctor Who* episode, or from the novel *The Day of the Triffids*. A desolate space, devoid of humanity, there are signs that people once lived here, but the inhabitants have long since gone. I didn't encounter a single cyclist on that final 10k stretch. I hardly saw a pedestrian either. The place was eerily vacant. The trees and the undergrowth looked normal, except that they were taking back possession of the cycle track, encroaching on both sides unchecked by any human passers by. The field of view is often restricted by earthen banks which rise on both sides of the Redway. Each leg of the track was unremittingly dull, looking exactly the same as the bit you had already covered. The tarmac surface was straight out of *The Day of the Triffids*, the bit where David takes his halftrack on a foraging mission along decayed, ruptured London streets, and a building collapses behind him, and he decides that it's no longer safe to be surrounded by man-made structures. That's where I was, a solitary runner, somewhere in the bleak, forsaken depths of Milton Keynes. The sound of road traffic was evident but the cars were usually hidden from sight behind earthen mounds, giving you only a rising and falling mechanical hum in the background. I was completely alone. At least *Doctor Who* had a travelling companion when he was stuck in strange worlds!

Alternating between running and walking, firstly switching at every 500m, then every 300m, and finally every 200m I yomped slowly towards The Dons' Stadium. Each time I slowed to a walk I checked my stopwatch, I did the mental arithmetic again, and I was cutting it really fine. Maybe on this 200m I need to try a bit harder? I'd run a little faster. Yes, that's OK. Don't ease off. Keep doing the maths. Keep yomping. You *cannot* afford to walk the whole of the remainder, you have to run some of it. And for goodness sake step up the pace when you run. Keep on keeping on as my friend Henry says!

There were no other runners in sight, neither ahead of me nor behind me. Fortunately there were no Triffids or Daleks either. And my stopwatch kept telling me that I was on target, but only just, and that I could do this. I was counting lampposts, measuring my progress in 100m chunks. Hoping that these lampposts were placed at the standard 100m distance. So even if I couldn't see waypoints in miles to guide my maths, I had lampposts to help me. And even if the lampposts were off plot, my ratio was correct, walk for two, run for two, I would effectively be running half of the remaining course.

In training I had only covered 33k once, and the theory goes that if you can do three quarter distance in training, then you can do the full distance on the day. In practice, my longer training runs were also examples of me yomping towards the end. Muscle fatigue played a part, but I don't remember that being a serious problem for me. The bigger battle was the psychological one. With more training, and a better strategy, I was thinking that I could have run the whole thing. I also knew that if the cut off time had been six hours, then I would have been perfectly able to summon up the mental strength and physical agility to meet that. And I wouldn't have rested at the humpback bridge for five minutes. And I would have adopted the sort of run walk run pattern that would get me to the finish in fractionally less than six hours.

I knew all this, and I knew I was taking liberties with myself and allowing myself the luxury of working to a longer cut off time. It was a mental battle, not a physical one. Here I was, now striving for a 6 hour 29 finish. The sweeper bus must be close by now. I scanned the distance behind me. There's nobody. There are no runners behind me because (I thought) they're probably already on the bus. But I still couldn't see a bus.

Just before the stadium, a long way ahead of me, I could make out the 26 Mile waypoint. The Redways were thankfully behind me, the road surface was now smooth tarmac, there was a smart concrete area outside the grandstand (where I had met the Stormtroopers), and I knew that awaiting me inside the stadium was a professionally tended 400m running track.

I also knew that the finish line was the regular finish line for the 100m sprint, and that I would run 300m of the 400m track to reach it. I looked at my watch. Run Paul! Run! Where I found the energy from I don't know, but the surface beneath my feet was now precisely what I needed, good solid hard material, and I began to smile. I passed the 26 Mile post. I left the road and joined the pavement. I was comfortable, I was on a good surface, and I was running at something like my normal pace. As I entered the stadium with 300m to go, my wife and my son were there cheering me on. So were two dozen other people.

If there was a sweeper bus it wasn't going to stop me now.

Inside the stadium I joined the back straight, checking my watch, just 300m left. As I reached the apex of that final curve, the clock above the finish line was already showing 6 hours 33. However, it's the chip time that counts, and my chip had been securely fastened to my shoe since I crossed the start line. The final 100m straight, another look at my watch, it assured me that I was OK.

Steady pace, no need for heroics now, no sprint. Thirty metres left, get ready, get that finger hovering over the button on the stopwatch. Hitting the stop button, plonking my foot on the sensor strip, I crossed the finish line, ecstatic, in 6 hrs, 28 mins 24 secs. I had completed my first marathon at 50 years of age, and I had beaten the sweeper bus by 96 seconds. I was placed 2,025 out of 2,046 and I had finished in a slightly better position than the one that John Backley advocated! I had fulfilled my objective.

I had *more than* fulfilled my objective. Back at the canal I had covered 600m more than the course required!

My family joined me briefly as I finished, congratulating me, and politely complaining that I had taken too long, and then they went back to the hotel.

There was no sweeper bus. I stayed inside the stadium and cheered on all the finishers who came in after me. There were 21 of them. They were all allowed to finish. I later learned that there had been more than 300 retirements. I suspect a few of them retired in the woods beyond that humpback bridge with the missing sign post!

Inside the stadium, the final runner crossed the line at 6 hrs 49 mins 31 secs, a veteran lady (age group 50 - 59) who finished with a bigger smile than I did. She was followed across the line by two paramedics on bicycles.

As I said earlier, I know that there are official photographers at these big events. By the time I reached the finish line they had already packed up and gone home. So had the water station, and the man handing out the free bananas. Soon after crossing the finish line I found a friendly race official who gave me a bottle of water, and the finishers' medal. She then opened up a big box of bananas and handed me one, I asked for another, and she said "you can have the whole box if you like" pointing behind her to a pallet stacked with about 20 boxes. If my car had been nearby I would have said yes, but I was on a bike that day. Moreover, I was planning to rest for a bit, have dinner in the hotel, rest a bit more, and then head home by train. I didn't feel that you could drag a big box of bananas into a Hilton Hotel, nor was it practical to leave it strapped onto a bike for two hours.

I went to the hotel, to the men's room where I changed my clothes, and then had dinner with the family. I was both elated and dejected in equal measure. Elated that I had completed a marathon. Dejected, because the event had been far removed from what I had expected. I had expected to be on a hard surface throughout, and totally segregated from the public. That's what you see on television when you watch the London Marathon or the Olympic Marathon. They only show you the nice bits. There's no entertainment value in showing you the pain and anguish and heartache on the worst bits of the course. Missing waypoints, missing signposts, decayed and ruptured surfaces, baby buggies blocking your way, hyped up sugar fuelled children disrupting everybody, and the detritus and neglected bits of the course that really belong in a science fiction novel.

You cannot really explain to an average runner (and I'm a very mediocre, average runner) what it's like to complete a marathon. You simply have to prepare for it the best you can, and then do it. I had been given so much anecdotal advice, but very little of it helped. I think that was because all of my advisors were young and fit twenty somethings or thirty somethings. I was an overweight 50 year old, running his first marathon! If you're not a serious runner you don't need the same advice as the serious enthusiasts. Go out and find a runner who's just like you. Ask them!

For me it wasn't a tough physical battle. I was carrying some excess weight (that's a handy supply of extra calories I thought), I shouldn't have consumed the energy gel the way I did, and I needed to take smaller amounts of water more often. Yes, I had some muscle fatigue during the race, but no cramp. What I genuinely did have to work hard on was the mental battle. The series of arguments between the part of the brain that wants to stop and the part that wants to keep going. In truth, I never seriously wanted to stop, I merely wanted to walk, and the other part of my brain wanted to run, and there was one crucial part of my brain overlording it over everything else, which said that I just wanted to finish before the sweeper bus. That overlordship won the day.

On 6 May 2013 in Milton Keynes I succeeded in joining the top *half of one per cent* of the UK population!

It was certainly not the experience that I had wanted, and that probably explains why it took me years before I was willing to try another marathon. To be honest, I had been thinking that one marathon was enough and I should call it quits.

The thought going through my head was "my distance is 10k and I should just stick to doing that".

Chapter 8 - A Modified Training Program

Falling off the wagon

Milton Keynes was over. The big target had been hit. Even if "only just" and although it was a resounding triumph, it was not the resounding triumph that I thought it might have been. I didn't go out running for a full four weeks after that race. When I finally decided to go out again, on Sunday 2 Jun 2013, I settled on an easy 8k run, a simple "out and back" with a loop of Battersea Park in the middle. Although before I had reached the 5k waypoint I managed to pull a muscle in my left heel. I walked, I ran, I walked, I yomped the last 3k home and I wished that I hadn't.

My log doesn't tell me if I did my stretches that day, but it does tell me that the muscle strain felt worse that evening and throughout the next day. For two weeks I used only the Tube to go to work, I didn't walk (Chapter 6 mentioned that I'd sometimes walk the 8k route to work) nor did I cycle. I was unhappy with the muscle strain, and I became annoyed with my old, stiff, work shoes. I threw them away and bought some Hush Puppies for the first time ever. Soft and supple. But that was a short lived experience. Within a few months the soles wore down quickly to a perfectly smooth glass like surface which was dangerous in wet weather, and especially dangerous on wet concrete steps. Think of Waterloo Bridge, or the many Tube station which have steps. By the end of 2013 I had gone back to wearing a new pair of my old, regular favourites, Clarks brogues.

In August 2013 I went on holiday for two weeks, and did no exercise. In effect, my enthusiasm for road running had waned in the middle of 2013 and by the time winter set in, I was unable to find the motivation to start running again. Inevitably an absence of training (mainly due to the absence of another big race to aim for) led to a gradual increase in my weight. By the end of 2015 the 12kg which I had lost throughout 2012 and 2013 had all returned! I needed to renew my campaign of health and fitness.

Moreover, it became abundantly clear to me that human beings were never designed to sit at a desk all day and work at a computer. I needed to build regular and significant exercise into my routine, or I was going to die prematurely from one or more lifestyle diseases linked to being overweight. At the end of 2015 my BMI was just over 30 again, clinically obese, and drastic action was needed.

Coincidentally, I picked up an interesting project after visiting some friends in Switzerland. For about three years from late 2015 to the summer of 2018 I worked concurrently in both London (my regular job) and in Switzerland (doing the education project). That meant that in early 2016 I was in Geneva when the adverts for the Geneva Marathon started to appear. In May 2016 I walked down to the lakeside to watch part of the event, ostensibly to cheer on the tail enders. The people like me! I had deliberately avoided the big, busy crowds that gather to watch the marathon at the height of the day.

Climbing back on the wagon

As I watched the marathon runners the bug bit me again. If I commit to running my second marathon, I thought, then surely I will have to train for it, and I will lose weight again! And this time, because it's my second marathon, I will know what I'm doing!

My project in Geneva was scheduled to end in early summer 2018. I hatched a plan. I could do some basic prep now. In 2016 I could enter one or more 10k races. In 2017 I could include one or two half marathons, one of which had to be the Geneva Half in May 2017. And in May 2018, before my project in Switzerland ended, I should be able to complete the Geneva Marathon.

Sorted! I had a general outline. It was nothing like a scientific plan, but I had more of a plan than I did last time. The Geneva Marathon 2018 was going to be a giant step up from Milton Keynes 2013. And I would be 55 years old by then.

In May 2016, with renewed enthusiasm, I started doing easy 6k routes twice a week. Although that had no effect on weight loss. I also looked around for races that I could enter which would fit my bizarre lifestyle spanning the UK and Switzerland. I developed two sets of training, Geneva during term time, and London during the school holidays.

I ended up with running routes in Troyes as well. If you drive the London Geneva route, an overnight stop in the middle of France shows that Troyes is perfect. And as my a long run was hard wired into my brain for Sunday mornings, all I had to do was head out early in Troyes and get back to the hotel in time to join my family in the dining room for breakfast, before the buffet stopped. I also visit Japan every year, and so I established several options for covering different distances in my adopted home city of Fukuoka.

None of that happened before marathon one.

If I was away from home, my running stopped. Now, when I prepared for my business trips and my holidays I also had to prepare to go running. No ifs, no buts. If I'm going to live a long and healthy life then I going to make *permanent* changes to the way I organise my life. Permanent features do not have to be modified when you're on a trip. It's the other way around, the trip's itinerary needs to be planned to accommodate the permanent features of your life.

At the end of 2016 my easy 6k route was increased to 10k, and instead of running it twice per week, I started running it three times per week. That kick started the new weight loss trend.

Remarkably, that also made things so much easier! The twice a week routine, meant one run on a Wednesday before work, and one run at the weekend. The change to doing it three times per week, meant every Tuesday, every Thursday and every Sunday. That pattern started on 1 Oct 2016 and (injuries permitting) continues to this day. It does vary a little depending on (a) adverse weather and (b) diary commitments. I found that the perfect running weather is 11°C with an overcast sky, or even the mildest possible drizzle. However, I'll also go out in various levels of bad weather as long as it's not absurd. In weeks when I have a long haul flight, I still try to put in three training runs, although the precise days may be vary from my standard pattern.

Running three times a week became normal, and it began to feel part of my usual routine, whereas running twice a week had felt like a chore and a disruption to my usual routine. I also invested in four sets of identical running kit, so that I never faced issues like "can't run today, laundry not done".

My training runs take place shortly after I wake up, and before I eat breakfast. I normally depart between 6.00am and 6.30am and that way I avoid the worst of any pedestrian traffic.

Fine Tuning the Wagon

I fell off the wagon, I climbed back on the wagon, and then I started fine tuning the wagon. I can summarise the differences like this:

Marathon One Training	Marathon Two Training
Inconsistent units, miles then kilometres	Everything in kilometres
Routes that fit the natural layout of the local roads	Routes established to match exactly 10k, 12k, etc
Routes measured on WalkJogRun.com	Routes measured by odometer
One or two runs per week	Three runs per week
Assorted bits of running kit	Four full sets of standardised attire
Large gaps in the training schedule	A transition to running every week
A mix of morning and evening runs	Always out running before breakfast
No running during holidays	Always running, even on holiday
New Balance running shoes	Nike Pegasus running shoes
Bum bag	Runners backpack

What this *before and after* table shows is that originally the approach to training had been a little ad hoc, whereas it had now become a bit more co-ordinated.

And as Chapter 3 explained, I had settled on using Nike Pegasus running shoes, because they felt comfortable, more like slippers than shoes.

I also invested in a runners backpack, but only after prompting by a friend, about two months before the Geneva Marathon 2018.

Measurement

In order to be sure that my distances were accurate I had also bought an odometer for my bike. I went out and measured (most of) my routes by cycling them. The fiddly bit with the bicycle odometer was calibrating it to match the circumference of my wheel. I went through the process about four times before I was happy with the accuracy. And I tested the accuracy against the odometer on my car using a straight eight kilometre stretch of road, driving and cycling that road twice in each direction. I double checked everything using the satellite view on the WalkJogRun website.

WalkJogRun was a really helpful website, maintained by two people who were both running enthusiasts and software developers. It was a work of passion for them and when it became really popular the workload overwhelmed them. The API drew data from Google Maps so I trusted the figures. However, the number of users on the site mushroomed! So many users registered and added routes that the hosts needed ever increasing amounts of data storage for routes, and they eventually shut it down. I used it for about four years and it was my "go to" solution when looking for accurate route details. It wasn't so much that the software developers were providing it for free, they could easily have charged us to cover the infrastructure costs and data storage needs, but it was the time involved in maintenance that was too great. They had day jobs too. The service stopped, the domain name lapsed and now WalkJogRun.com is a completely different operation.

I don't like mobile apps. I don't like too little data on too small a screen. Nor do I want to give lots of personal information to the big corporates. The old version of WalkJogRun.com wanted a username and password only, and let me generate and store my maps without data mining them. I have found nothing else to match that.

I see that some of the organisers of races have used MapMyRun.com and plotaroute.com. The routes have been visible to all, until they aren't. Before one of my holidays travelling around Scotland I checked MapMyRun.com and I found a nice half marathon route in Cumbernauld. An overnight stop in Cumbernauld was duly scheduled for that week. On the Saturday when I arrived, the online route had been removed from the website. I used Google maps instead to hastily come up with a 10k route, and on the Sunday morning I ran that bit of Cumbernauld instead.

Late 2016 and Early 2017

By late 2016 my schedule looked like this:

- Weekly - 3 training runs
- Sunday - runs to incrementally increase to 20k by 30 Apr 2017
- 7 May 2017 - Geneva Half Marathon

Late 2017 and Early 2018

The intensity then increased:

- 8 Jul 2017 - the Sunday 10k incremented to 12k
- August onwards - once per month do an extra longer run, adding 2k each month
- Join the Geneva Runners meet up on every Saturday morning
- 6 May 2018 - Geneva Marathon

My distances steadily increased. I was away for a weekend in Leeds for a tech sector conference, and I took time out on Sunday 22 Apr 2018 to run my own half marathon course from the city centre to the edge of Rawdon, past Horsforth Golf Club, and back again.

By April 2018 I had reached a Sunday distance of 30k. Generally doing my standard 12k and my extended 30k on alternate Sundays. I went to Geneva Runners a number of times. Nice friendly people, but I was old, and I was still a slow outsider who never quite fitted in. Running with them mid morning on a Saturday didn't fit my routine and although they have evening runs too (on weekdays) those were never going to fit into my diary. What I did learn from the coffee and chat afterwards, is that investing in a runners backpack is well worth the money (as discussed in Chapter 2).

I can also see that a number of the members benefitted from having a "running buddy". Perhaps you can too. At my age, my pace, and my ability, my companions were doing their best to help me, but I always felt that I was holding them back. I'm sure the ideal "running buddy" exists for everyone. I'm not sure they're that easy to find.

The other thing that happened during 2017 and 2018 (when Twitter was still a reasonably useful website) was "Pick up the pace Paul". I had been active on

Twitter since 2008 and had established some good dialogue with other runners, one of whom was "Pick up the pace Paul". He was passionate about running marathons as the four hour pace setter. Sometimes he would agree a different figure, but guiding the "4 hour bus" was his favourite. He did many marathons across the UK and Europe, and I remember seeing him discuss guiding one of them in Cyprus.

I lost touch with him after I abandoned Twitter at the end of 2021 by which time the site had largely turned into a toxic swamp.

However, Paul had shared so many stories from the pace setter point of view, that I parked the idea in my head that I might benefit from the help of a pace setter. Paul had also shown examples of the pace sheet worn on the opposite wrist from his watch. That was another idea that I might use.

On the last weekend before the Geneva Marathon, I cycled the marathon route on the Saturday, and my Sunday training run was an extended version of my local one, bringing the distance to 35k. With my longer training runs I had a figure of 8 arrangement taking me across the Switzerland/France border four times on a single run. Passing through the one at CERN, the two minor crossings at *Mategnin* (the one on the road rarely staffed, and the one of the footpath almost never staffed) and the big one at the *Ferney Voltaire* end of Geneva airport. The first couple of times I did that I carried my passport in my bum bag. I was never stopped. For all the later ones I took to carrying just my driving licence (for ID) and I never needed that either. In spite of the Brexit vote in 2016, the Schengen rules still applied to Brits traversing borders, and the *gendarmes* showed no interest in an old man crossing the border in running kit.

The training programme for Geneva involved a lot more running, and longer distances than before. In Geneva, London, and elsewhere. Some of the longer runs were a little boring so I developed interesting mind games to keep myself occupied. One of which was to invent personas for some of the people I saw. Mr Grim and Mr Last Orders were the ones who initiated this amusing habit. Some of them I saw only once. I saw The Harlem Shuffler many times.

Real Life Semi Fictional Characters

Mr Grim — Short for grimace, he looks like Sisyphus pushing a ball up a hill, puffing, panting, and groaning, but there's no ball, and there's no hill. In spite of which, he's still trying to run and groan at the same time.

Mr Last Orders	He's a fat fellow who runs like a bulldog using short quick mini steps, as if he desperately has to get to the bar before the end of last orders.
The Windmill	With every stride his arms seem do more work than they have to. Yes, you can swing your arms to promote a faster run, but Mr Windmill still manages to do that twice as much as he needs to.
Mr Fog Horn	With every stride he emits a noise, in tune with his breathing, repeatedly doing three soft sounds and then one long blast on the fog horn: *hah hah hah HARHHHH*
Mr Orgasm	With every stride he emits a noise. That's all I'm telling you. Use your imagination!
The Little Drummer Boy	How noisy can one man's feet be? Lots of short steps, each one striking the ground with a smart drum beat. Perhaps he can cope with the noise because he's wearing ear plugs?
The Harlem Shuffler	Remarkable running style type 1 - a lovely old man, his feet barely leave the ground, and each arm moves in a unique pattern. An unbalanced gait, in spite of which he runs at a reasonable pace, and is intriguing to watch.
Miss Mis-Step	Remarkable running style type 2 - maybe she's double jointed? At every step her feet rise, her toes go up and sideways, and her ankles remain on track. Perhaps she pronates uniquely? It's amazing to see each foot return to the ground correctly, and enable her to continue running.
Miss Tulip Tip Toe	Remarkable running style type 3 - you have to do a double take to make sure this is for real. Her heels never touch the ground. It looks like she could easily tip toe through the tulips.
Miss Wobble Bottom	Self explanatory. She's big enough to be two people but she's only one. It's admirable that she's out jogging slowly. Maybe start with some walking?
Mr DFT	He's a big chap, he approaches you with all the speed and grace of a *derailed freight train* going sideways, so don't stand in his way!
Mr Happy	That's me!

Before the Geneva Half Marathon in 2017 I had cycled the 21k route. In 2018 I cycled the full marathon route. Having been shocked by some of the surfaces in Milton Keynes, I wanted to know exactly what I was letting myself in for prior to doing the races in Geneva. I'm not used to cycling 66k on a Brompton folding bike with a hard seat, but I had to cover 14 + 42 + 10 on Saturday 28 Apr 2018. My rear end was sore for three days, but it was fine by the day of the race.

The surfaces were largely a mix of major and minor roads, with decent tarmac. Somewhere near *Pont de la Motte* there was a short stretch of farm track, perhaps 300m, made of rough cast concrete covered with stones and detritus chucked up by tractors. Elsewhere there was good quality block paving for some footpaths, and very occasionally a stretch of rough gravel, where some semi-rural footpaths running off to at 90° to the road had not been perfectly connected at the kerb. In other places, block paving and gravel were laid side by side in an odd 50/50 arrangement.

The Geneva course was far better than Milton Keynes. And more importantly, I had advance knowledge of where the defects were, how bad they were, and how far I had to run on them. Basically there were *some* defects and they were all negligible. There were no grassy bits and no humpback bridges!

Back on the day of the Geneva Half Marathon in 2017 there had been some rain the preceding night, and the course was flooded at about the 7k point. It was on a narrow, winding country road near *Choulex*, and it flooded for a distance of about 80 metres, to a depth of about 10cm. Not a problem if you were in a car or on a bike.

We were on foot. Around half of the runners elected to run through the water, and clearly had wet feet for the rest of the race. Along with the other half, I decided to avoid the flood by treading carefully through a wet muddy field and emerging beyond the water. Then I tried to wipe the soles of my shoes on the wet muddy grass verge, the same as many others, before I resumed my race with mercifully intact, dry socks and feet.

The Black Belt in Karate

My self managed training program requires me to enter official races every so often. I did my third *half marathon* in early 2017, and completed that one in 2 hrs 28 mins 36 secs. A new personal best! So the older I get, the faster I get! That's a trend that can't last?

> I also ran a personal best in a 10k race in August 2017 achieving 59 mins 5 secs, and since then I bettered even that. On my 10k training run on 28 Sep 2017, I managed 56 mins 23 secs. I put that down to perfect running weather, a temperature of 12°C, and perfect mindset that morning.
>
> Those times are not especially impressive. Though I'm not really judging myself against the rest of the runners I meet, but against my younger self.
>
> That's what a Grand Master 14th Dan black belt in Karate does! There is nobody else at 14th Dan black belt, so he can only compete against his younger self. Using a points based system, his performance is judged by his peers.
>
> By 2017, 54 year old Paul was beating 44 year old Paul at everything!

There's a positive self reinforcing feedback loop at work in my training. The more I run, the more I lose weight, and the better my times become. Likewise, the faster I run, the fitter I become, and the more weight I lose. Between January and October 2017 my BMI went from 30.7 to 27.1, and I was well happy!

I aimed to complete my second marathon in about 5 hours 30 mins. At that time I was sure that 55 year old Paul could beat 50 year old Paul (6 hours 28 mins) and in any case, the Geneva sweeper bus operated at 6 hours, so I had to beat 6 hours! To be honest, I was thinking that I could do it in about 5 hours.

Based on the longer runs at the end of 2017 I was even thinking that it could be a bit quicker than that, estimating 4 hours 48 mins with my own spreadsheet model. Anyway, common sense says "aim for 5 hours 30 and that'll be one hour better than last time!"

Knowing that around one half of one per cent of the UK population has completed a marathon, I now want to know what percentage of the UK population has completed two marathons? Can you help me find that data? Because I can't!

Chapter 9 - Marathon 2 Geneva

Sunday 6 May 2018

Normally I don't eat breakfast on a Sunday morning before I go out for a run. However, the start time for the marathon was 9.45am and I was up as usual at around 5.30am. So, for breakfast I had one banana, and probably three cups of tea! Enough to sustain me on my journey to *Chêne-Bourg* some 12k from where I lived.

I checked the forecast online and went outside to double check. A lovely warm pleasant morning, a cloudless sky, and a light wind. The temperature at 5.30 was already 14°C and it was due to rise to about 26° by mid afternoon.

Due to the light wind I decided that needed a long sleeved top. Both to travel to and from the race, and to keep me sufficiently warm right up to the moment that the race started. It wasn't going into the bag drop! I selected my nicest, most comfortable long sleeved top, and I would need to wear it or carry it for the whole day. I also decided that tracksuit trousers would be a good idea for the commute. I had prepared all of this kit the night before, and waited for the morning before deciding precisely what I would wear.

There were 9,000 entries for Geneva Marathon in 2018, and we all had free passes to ride Geneva's public transport for the whole day. The start was at *Chêne-Bourg* about 4k south of the finish on *Pont du Mont Blanc*, which is right in the middle of the city centre. My family spent more than 6 hours waiting for me to complete the Milton Keynes Marathon in 2013 so this time they opted to stay at home. In the early days they'd come along and give me moral support. After seven years of repeatedly doing various races, they justifiably left me to it. After all, a second marathon is not as special as the first!

Without them around, I would need to use the bag drop facility. I had a change of socks and a T shirt ready, a small towel, my everyday trainers, and a bottle of water packed into a small draw string bag. Although I rarely travelled south of *Rive* I knew Geneva's tram routes well, and I had been to *Chêne-Bourg* a handful of times. I wanted to reach the start long before thousands of runners clogged up the transport system, and especially because there was no way to avoid a change of trams in the city centre.

Extra trams and buses had been laid on, but I still wanted to be early. The plan was to have plenty of time to find the bag drop, find a toilet, do all my stretches, and look for the 5 hour pace setter. I wanted to have a brief chat with the pace setter, I wanted to do that accurately in English, and had revised enough French vocab in case I needed that.

Living on the extreme north side of the city the buses on Sunday mornings were few and far between. To be certain of getting an early tram I walked a fair distance to the first/last stop. When it set off I was the only runner on board, amongst five or six other passengers. Gradually it filled up, lots of us already wearing our bibs, and smiling politely at one another. In the city centre there's a big intersection at *Bel Air* where several tram lines converge. Along with hundreds of other runners I slowly walked the 150m from *Bel Air* to *Molard* to join the next tram. The place was already heaving at 8.30am. I wouldn't have liked to have left it any later. There was no space to get onto the first tram at *Molard* though I was able to squeeze onto the next one. Tightly packed like sardines we were all going 4k south to *Chêne-Bourg*.

The area around the start was closed off to regular traffic. The tram arrived (at its final stop) at about 9.00am, which left me a good 45 minutes to get myself organised. I walked around to familiarise myself with the facilities. There were already modest queues for the portaloos, so I took the chance to immediately join the queue and use one. A wait of just a few minutes. After that, I applied sun cream everywhere, to the back of my neck and ears, all over my face, and paid particular attention to the increasingly large bald patch on the top of my head.

I checked where the 5 hour start pen was, and I noticed that the pace setter was busy chatting in his native French to a group of about five female runners. The nearby bag drop was arranged in two large trucks. I removed my tracksuit trousers, added them to my bag, along with the remains of my sun cream, and I handed the bag in.

As planned, I was still wearing my favourite long sleeved top. The wind was light, but I was glad to have my top. I intended removing the top at about 2k. Potentially that meant that I would have to transfer my bib from that top to my T shirt and honestly, I didn't want the hassle. Hence, I put my long sleeved top on first, and wore my T shirt over it, with the bib fixed firmly to the shirt by four safety pins. This meant that a brief stop was needed where I would remove two tops, and then put the T shirt back on again. The long sleeved top would then be tightly folded and would (just) fit into the large pocket at the rear of my backpack, jammed in with the water bladder. I didn't want to discard my favourite long sleeved top so I had no option but to carry it for the race.

The forecast was for hot and sunny weather, and that's what my baseball cap is for. When the sun is shining in the most awkward way, the cap keeps it out of my eyes. The rest of the time I allow my head to sweat freely, putting the whole surface area to work, and letting the sweat band do its job. I rely on sun cream to keep me safe.

With around 20 minutes to go, I completed my stretches routine and made my way over to the 5 hour pen. And then I decided that I wanted the toilet again! The portaloo queues were massive. The most suitable hedgerow was obvious by the collection of other male runners who were one step ahead of me. I probably wouldn't need the toilet again until the finish. I then headed to the 5 hour pen and made a direct line for the pace setter, introduced myself, and in the best French I could muster I explained it was my second marathon and . . .

Mr Grumpy wasn't interested. Either he had already had enough newbies to deal with that morning, or my French was worse than I thought, or he simply wrote me off as a time waster the moment I said *"deuxième marathon"*. With 15 minutes remaining before the start I had established no rapport, and I decided that it was up to me to manage my own running.

The modern disco music on the public address system was too loud, and not to my liking, the warm up guy with the microphone was over excited, interposing some English in his French, and the runners were jumping up and down (except for me), cheering and waving (I managed a brief dignified wave) as a small drone from the TV station passed overhead. The 5 hour pen was probably a good 800m from the start line. We heard the starting pistol, we heard the cheers from the crowd, and we knew that the elite runners had set off.

My group didn't move. We didn't budge one centimetre. Although judging by their repressed movement a lot of people around me had evidently expected to be mobile instantly. It took time. A short wait, a bit of a shuffle, a geriatric walk, then a slow walk, a bit faster, and by the time we'd covered the 800m to the start line we had a slow jog under way. Dutifully plonking my foot on the sensor, I crossed the start line and started my stopwatch.

All the runners around me zoomed off like a shot. That surprised me. I was aiming for a 5 hour pace, and in my book that meant consistency from start to finish. That probably upset the runner directly behind me who had clearly expected me to run faster and conform to the peer pressure. I was conforming to nothing, other than my own plan!

As with Milton Keynes I struggled to find my stride at the start. Even at my slower pace I was going faster than I wanted to, because I was trying to avoid collisions with other runners. The pack thinned out a bit, and by 500m I had a little personal space and I tried to settle into my comfort zone. Just ahead of me a young man stepped off the road, onto the pavement, ran across the grass, and up to the bushes. Clearly a toilet break! I wonder if he'd planned that all along or if the portaloo queues had simply proven too intimidating?

At one kilometre, the waypoint was in exactly the right place. So was the 2k waypoint. I was happy about that. I was slightly ahead of schedule and I was running through a hospital car park! Hang on! A hospital car park? I had glanced upwards to look at the 2k sign at the side of the road, then I looked down at my stopwatch, and when I looked up again I was now running between two rows of parked cars! We all were. OK, so I'm obviously still on the same route as everybody else! I hope there's an exit straight ahead of me because I don't want to be doing any sharp 90° turns inside a tightly packed car park. Predictably the exit was where it should be.

This bit of the course was the same as last year (when I did the half marathon) and I wondered if I had been paying much attention back then. I didn't remember a car park! I had no recollection of anything hindering me at this stage in the 2017 half marathon.

We were still a bit bunched up in the car park, after which the runners started thinning out some more. We did a gentle 90° right turn onto a local country road, followed by another comfortable 90° turn to the left, and then we were on our way into some proper countryside. By now I had some space to myself and it wasn't long before I found my stride and settled into a comfortable pace.

The 3k waypoint came into view. I should be removing my long sleeved top now. For the benefit of the runners behind me I signalled that I was moving off the road, and stopped on the cyclepath. Where I partially undressed (to a chorus of cheers from the other runners), stowed my long sleeved top, restored my T shirt and backpack to their proper places, and continued. Comfortable! Both with my clothing and with my newly found pace. I was a little ahead of schedule, ahead of the 5 hour pace setter, and even though I was faster than intended I decided to settle like this, looking for "flow".

By my reckoning 80% of the runners were ahead of me. The over enthusiastic part of the "five hour pen" were also ahead of me, and the pragmatists were somewhere behind me clustered around Mr Grumpy. I had no obvious cohort to run with, so I was already "on my own" in that sense, with the occasional runner overtaking me. I also clearly recognised these roads. The first 7k of the marathon course was the same route that I had followed the year before when I did the half. Funny that I didn't remember running through a hospital car park though! Then I recalled that the road had split in two, and you could have run around either side of the hospital to get to the same place. This year I had naturally gone with the flow of runners going to the left. The year before I had presumably gone to the right.

There was a lot of good quality tarmac as I moved off one road turning left onto another. And recalling last year's half marathon, and last week's cycle around the route, I knew that the first water station wasn't far away. It was beside that path with the mixed surface where I could choose to run on the gravel bit or the block paving. Whilst doing all this mental mapping in my head I had not seen much happening in my peripheral vision. Until I was almost upon them.

There were two men to my right, in a ditch, both clearly paramedics. They were bent forwards, their backs facing me, and I didn't really see the casualty. For the merest fraction of a second I caught sight of a runner who had ended up in the ditch. Men's clothing, hairy legs, and - and then I was past them - I didn't clock the runner's stature or age, simply that he was completely immobile, not one muscle moving at all. This was between 5k and 6k. Whether he was young or old, forced off the road, or suffered dehydration, or some kind of seizure, I could only speculate.

No other runners or spectators were there, just the two paramedics and one casualty. I've seen casualties at races before. I've never before (nor since) seen one who was unconscious, nor have I ever seen one as early at 6k into a race. They're usually at the roadside in the second half of a race, limping, clutching their leg, or getting a massage from a suitably skilled member of the volunteer team.

This stationary casualty preyed on my mind a little and I reminded myself of my own golden rules for running. Starting with the morbid "you're trying to live longer, not kill yourself". I only have to beat the sweeper bus, I don't need to beat 5 hours, and to be honest if I have to retire from the race I will retire. It's OK to not be OK.

I approached the first water station, I didn't need to stop, and I took a couple of sips from my own supply. I have no idea how and when dehydration sets in, but as a minimum I will take (my own) water every time I pass a water station. Naturally, I will also take water at any other interval I like, because I'm wearing my new backpack. If I happen to empty it, then I will stop and refill it at the next available water station. No matter how hot it gets today I will not suffer dehydration. What I didn't know in advance was that most (if not all) of the water stations also provided runners with segments of orange. At the first water station I missed the opportunity to pick up one or two pieces, and I didn't want to turn back.

We were deep into Swiss countryside now, and I recognised the road that had been flooded last year. Perfectly dry this time, and no need for a detour through a wet muddy field. These small back roads are not great, but if I run along the middle of the road I'm not affected by the camber, and the road surface is also better. Some of those roads were low grade, resembling farm tracks and a few had a fair sprinkling of gravel and other small stones. Especially the bit where the marathon course goes right and the half marathon course goes left. This concrete farm track was new territory for me. Yes, I did cycle it "last week", but I had never actually run on this route before, and this surface is a tiny bit tedious. My speed went down, my eyes fixated on where I was placing each foot, and 300m of ultra cautious running ensued. Fortunately it was only 300m, and I was back on a rudimentary country road formed of adequate tarmac. Of the entire course, only that 300m (at around 8k) gave me any cause for concern. Far, far better than the Milton Keynes experience.

Avoiding the mistake I had previously made, taking excess water and energy gel, this time I had brought my own boiled sweets along. One each as I completed each quarter of the course. Approaching the 10k waypoint I took one, quickly crushing it with teeth, swallowing it all, and rinsing my mouth with water from my backpack. It was a sugar boost.

As we ran up to the llama farm I was joined by two young men from Manchester, one was reasonably athletic and experienced, and was theoretically helping his stocky, overweight friend to run his first marathon. We ran together for a good 2k and it was clear that the experienced man wanted to make better progress, and that the larger man had underestimated what running a marathon involved. The sun was higher, the temperature was up and he was flagging. This was at about the 10k to 12k stage, not even half way. It wasn't said but it was unmistakably implied that 30 year old Mr Stocky should tag along with 55 year old me at my pace, and young Mr Experience would head off at his regular pace.

That's what happened . . . until about 15k when Mr Stocky kindly told me to carry on, and he would walk. He could now envision a 6 hour finish, according to his calculations, just by walking, and he would narrowly avoid the sweeper bus. I wished him well as I reached the top of a gentle ascent, heading towards the forest in the near distance.

By now, I was happy with my pace, my time, and periodically I was passing one or two of the other runners. They all seemed younger than me, and I was thinking they had made the mistake of setting off too fast and suffering the consequences too soon. By 16k it was clear that most of the runners I was passing were less experienced, and were not particularly well prepared. Sometimes I would have a running partner for a few hundred metres, but these liaisons were brief and none of us were a perfect match for the other.

At one point I caught up with a young British Indian girl who was struggling to run and take a selfie at the same time. Following a brief conversation I agreed to simply stop for 30 seconds or so, stage the photo opportunity, be the photographer and get that "proof" that she so wanted to share. Vantage point and running space were quickly established, using her phone I took 4 or 5 shots, she checked them, was thoroughly delighted, and we resumed running.

Once more, I was the old man running faster than the younger entrant. I say "faster" but it wasn't fast really! Just relative to the others I was having a better time of it. It was certainly hot. The sun was higher, though I felt prepared and in control.

I was confident that I could do the distance. Now I only had to focus on managing the pace and aiming for a sensible time. At the water station at 17k I was really happy and was convinced that I could better 5 hours. That particular water station not only had segments of orange, but also chunks of banana. And children aged 8 or 9 handing out the fruit.

I had time to exchange only a couple of sentences with them as I accepted both orange and banana, telling them how delighted I was that they had made the effort to turn out to bring *me* fruit, especially *me*, because *j'adore bananes*. Getting very brief interactions with marshals, spectators and volunteers is a great morale booster for me. If a spectator is cheering, clapping, and looking at me with eye contact I will always respond, usually with something like *"vous êtes mon ami"*. Whether it has the same impact as *"you're my friend"* said in English I don't know, but we both leave the encounter all the richer for it.

I had barely finished my orange and banana when I reached the small fire station on the edge of the village. Thoughtfully *les sapeurs pompiers* had rigged up a watering facility like a shower. Imagine a professional gardener with a powerful hose with an adjustable spray head for watering plants, something like that, only on a more serious scale. Pointed upwards it provided a broad expanse of artificial light rain across the entire road, and the *sapeur* holding the device could give you more or less of a drenching. I watched runners ahead of me deliberately move left to avail themselves of more of the cold shower. However, I detest running in wet socks and shoes, and so I veered right. The look of horror on my face probably said more than my French skills could ever convey, and *Monsieur Sapeur* obligingly pointed the spray at the field behind him and not above the road. As I passed him we smiled at each other knowingly. I'm sure I wasn't the first runner like that.

Further down beyond the village of *Jussy*, near the French border by *Annemasse Saint-Cergues*, there are wide expanses of rural Switzerland which have all the attraction of Norfolk. Barren, dull and flat. I plodded on, only now beginning to feel the heat, and a bit of fatigue. And a bit of boredom. On this stretch I dutifully consumed one more boiled sweet as I passed the 20k waypoint. This *back of beyond* bit of the course was the only bit which was featureless, save for the odd collection of a few trees set far back from the road. It was also the only place where the closed roads were not "closed". At least that was I thought after two cars emerged from a farm house and gingerly crawled down the road to pass me.

The emptiness of the surroundings compounded the boredom, and my train of thought focussed on fatigue. I was on my own. At one remote crossroads there was one marshal directing runners. He was sheltered from the sun inside his car, which was parked under a large gazebo. His car window was down, the radio was loud and he was obviously bored too. A long way ahead of me there were two runners. And some considerable distance behind me there was one more. There was no sign at the midpoint, but we all knew (in metric) that the midpoint is 97.5 metres after the 21k waypoint. I judged that I hit the midpoint at 2 hours 20 comfortably ahead of my target, and so I reasoned that a time of 4 hours 40 was theoretically possible. But I also knew that my pace was beginning to slow. I still thought that 5 hours was possible as long as I was diligent about my pace in the second half.

As I approached the edge of the city again some buildings came into sight. First the village of *Presinge* and then *Puplinge*. They signalled a return to normality. Having skirted around *Jussy* on the dispiriting and empty minor roads, seeing some people again helped stimulate my brain. Not spectators as such, but welcome human beings nonetheless. The polite smiles, waves and occasional shouts of "*allez allez allez*" cheered me up a little.

The French gendarmes had joined the Swiss gendarmes watching the road from the Swiss side. As I ran within a few metres of the border crossing at *Annemasse* they shouted encouragement. I turned right onto *Route de Cornière* leading into the village of *Puplinge* proper. As soon as I passed the boundary sign at the edge of the village I abruptly changed from a run to a walk.

That wasn't planned.

Compared to Milton Keynes where my walking had started immediately after the midpoint, I was pleased that I had at least run a bit further this time. In Geneva I unintentionally resorted to walking at about 24.7k. I walked for 300m to the sign at the 25k waypoint, and then I picked up the pace again.

What had been the problem? Aching legs. Rather surprised! Aching legs already? Especially my calf muscles. I couldn't recall that being as early as 25k on my training runs, but perhaps it was. I knew it was coming at some stage and

I had been hoping that I could get a fair bit further before feeling too much pain. I thought to myself, in future I have to write more comprehensive notes about my training runs. A big mental debate was starting in my head. How was I going to manage the remaining 17k of this course, and what would my revised target time be?

Yomping was my solution.

In the time that it took me to travel 1,200m from one side of *Puplinge* to the other I had pretty much committed to yomping the whole of the remaining course. I had now passed the 26k waypoint. I toyed with the idea of slowing for 10 or 20 minutes (or however long it would take) for Mr Grumpy to catch up with me, and then tag on to his 5 hour bus. Yes, a questionable strategy I thought, and I decided to defer making that decision until he drew alongside me at some point further along the course.

If I was going to join the 5 hour bus then I would be committed to running at his pace for at least the final 10k. I wasn't sure if I wanted to stomach that. It would deprive me of my yomping tactic. And I was certain that if I yomped while artificially matching the 5 hour bus, alternating my walking and my running, repeatedly passing them and being passed by them, it would wind him up even more (and all of his cohort). I reasoned that joining the 5 hour bus was a sure fire recipe to make all of us feel grumpy.

The decision making moment came a lot sooner than I expected. I was on the bit of the course leading to *Choulex*, the bit "in the middle" of the figure 8 course where the runners cover the same 4k for a second time. The water station at the 6k waypoint is also roughly the 27.5k mark. Before reaching the water station, Mr Grumpy passed me. I was walking at the time, he had a bus of about four people, and I was in no position to start running to keep up with them. The decision had been made by my legs not my brain.

To boot, I now knew that I was not going to better five hours, because the 5 hour bus had passed. I needed to double down on my yomping strategy, determined to beat the sweeper bus at six hours. This was Milton Keynes all over again. Except it wasn't. I was much better prepared. I was sipping tiny bits of water when I wanted it. No excess fluids were slopping around inside me. No energy gel, but boiled sweets instead. I was also a second time marathoner.

And I knew this course. The remaining surface was good. Having run the half marathon the year before, and having cycled the whole course the week before, I knew that the final 10k meant top quality tarmac on major roads leading into and around the city.

So I knew what was in store for me, and I also knew that I had the ability to complete a marathon, because I'd done one before. I would simply have to do the mental arithmetic repeatedly, and keep on keeping on. If I could do 6 hours 28 ahead of a 6 hour 30 cut off in Milton Keynes, then I could do 5 hours 58 ahead of Geneva's 6 hour cut off.

My legs hurt. My brain didn't. If anything the novice running experience and my knowledge of the course, combined with my reworked plan, put me in a better frame of mind. I was now a lot more cheerful than I was when I passed the bored marshal in the middle of Norfolk style Switzerland.

At about 30k I consumed one more sweet. By which time the British Asian girl had caught up with me, chatted briefly, and passed me.

"Are you OK?"
"Yes, I'm fine. I can finish. Just a bit too hot for me, that's all."
"Best of luck!"

And she slowly progressed ahead of me. I didn't want to say "my legs hurt" because at that stage of a marathon everybody's legs hurt. I thought that "it's a bit too hot" was a diplomatic way to explain my reduced performance without interfering with her determination to run in spite her own achy legs.

A British couple ahead of me were also walking. It took me a little time, but I caught up with them. They looked at my attire. The sweatband on my head always makes me stand out. It also deceives people into thinking that I'm a more advanced runner than I really am.

This young husband and wife couple wanted me to tell them about the timing on *my* stopwatch. Like me, their adjusted plan was to beat the sweeper bus, though back in the excitement of the start line they had failed to start either of their stopwatches until much later. Hence, they weren't able to make exact calculations and were fearful of now being too slow. Nor did they want to tag on to me and yomp the remaining course. They were firmly committed to power walking it. He left his watch running with his current timing. She restarted her stopwatch based on my explanation that we had about 80 minutes remaining.

Obviously they hadn't crossed the start line at exactly the same time as me, but the new information helped them feel a lot happier. What I did learn from them, because he was wearing a really fancy, modern watch, was that the afternoon temperature had now reached 30°. That news didn't make me feel any happier, but it did eliminate any guesswork. Everybody was burdened by the heat. Except for the fastest runners who had already finished!

The descent towards the lake starts above the village of *Collonge-Bellerive* and takes you through a tunnel beneath the centre of the village. A major road tunnel, no sunshine, cool air (relatively speaking), impeccable tarmac, a gentle descent, and bliss. Achy legs actually, so not really bliss, but it's the nearest thing you're going to get to bliss at the 34k to 35k stage. And so, inside this road tunnel I ran. Although it might have been tempting to stay in the tunnel for longer, I went through it as fast as my legs would carry me. Given the condition I was in, it was my last opportunity to make good progress at my regular running speed, using the comfortable environment to its max.

Back into the sunshine, the *Jet d'Eau* was now visible, with the city of Geneva as a back drop. What's that odd feeling? My shoes have suddenly become tighter! Could it have been a result of the transition from the cool dark tunnel to the bright warm sunshine? No! Extra heat would have caused the shoes to expand not contract. Had my feet expanded? No idea! My size 7 shoes were perhaps not the right ones for me. I parked that thought in my head and resolved to buy size 7.5 shoes before my next major run. In any case, the squeeze created only the tiniest hint of discomfort for my feet, but nothing like the persistent pain in my lower legs.

I went into what I call my "classic" yomping mode. I was on a long gentle descent lasting about 4k. Yomp! Run for two lampposts, walk for two lampposts. By now there were rarely any runners overtaking me. But I was passing some of those ahead. The 35k waypoint. Just over 7k left, and I had 56 minutes left. Even Mr Grumpy and his 5 hour bus had finished by now. It was stupidly hot, my legs were killing me. OK, obviously they weren't literally killing me, but that conveys the pain, and that's the vernacular that English speakers use.

A Japanese entrant was ahead of me, somewhere near *Bébé Plage*, he was walking with a merest hint of a limp, but he was still on the move, and (by my reckoning) was still in with a chance of beating the sweeper bus. I knew he was Japanese because people who wear a head band in that fashion are a common sight in Japan. Not a terylene sweatband like mine, but a strip of cotton cloth wrapped around the head and knotted at the back. As I drew closer it was clear from the writing on the back of his T shirt that he was Japanese. I slowed down to his pace and walked beside him. He was about ten years younger than me, in his mid forties, a pained expression on his face, and then an astonished expression as I spoke to him in natural Japanese. Urging him to "*ganbarimasho ne*", to keep up the effort, telling him that he could complete this course, he had enough time, he just needed to persevere and keep on keeping on.

Now at the south eastern edge of Geneva I was on very familiar ground, the spectators were out in force, the alpine cow bells they ring were loud and annoying. But in any case, I was grateful for any encouragement, and anything that took my mind off the pain in my calf muscles. I was 4k from the finish. I could see it, because I would be passing close to the finish line (which was southbound on one bridge) as I crossed northbound on another bridge, then loop through the city centre, head north east for a bit, do a wide U turn at *Parc Mon Repos* and then join the final stretch down to *Pont du Mont Blanc*.

Not only were there spectators everywhere, there was a fair assortment of runners who had already finished and were now walking home. Entrants in their running kit, with their marathon bibs, and proudly sporting their finisher medals. As I passed the 38k waypoint I could see all this. I checked my watch. I was going to finish, I was going to have one of those medals, and my mental arithmetic was telling me that I should finish comfortably within 6 hours.

I went north over the narrow bridge, the *Pont des Bergues*, where last year a marshal had spotted the UK flag on my bib and had shouted at me in English "you can do this". She wasn't there this year, so subconsciously I shouted in my head "you can do this" and I smiled warmly to myself. And I knew I could do it. The pain in my legs was now a standard feature that I had learned to accept, the 30° heat was just about tolerable too. At every water station in the latter half of the race I had been taking tiny amounts of the water and a segment of orange. That had enabled me to preserve the water in my backpack and make it last to the end. Equally important to me, I was running on perfectly level ground beside the lake, and the road surface was good.

The Geneva Marathon is a nice marathon. So much better than running on the Redways in the closing stages of the Milton Keynes Marathon. Geneva had none of the repeated ascents and descents which had bugged me last time (the bridges and subways which pass through the roundabouts).

Best of all, I was going to finish for sure, and I was on for a record time. OK, this was only my second marathon, but I was looking for every reason I could find to be cheerful. I was going to beat my (relatively easy to beat) personal best of 6 hours 28. I was now on track for 5 hours 50 something - low fifties - so I was definitely on track and I had some time to spare!

Skirting around the edge of *Cornavin* where the main railway station is located, I followed a mix of major and minor roads which lead onto the broad, lakeside boulevards, first *Quai du Mont Blanc* and then *Quai Wilson*. I passed *Bains des Pâquis* where these two major roads meet. It's the place where people can swim in the lake, and it's the place where the Geneva Runners meet up on Saturday mornings. I looked towards the coffee shop, saw nobody I recognised, and I imagined that they'd either be down near the finish line, or more likely they'd all have gone home by now.

A good turnout of spectators had conscientiously chosen to remain near the finish throughout the later stages of the race. I wanted to demonstrate that I was putting in a conscientious effort too. Time for some modified yomping, change the ratio, run for four lampposts, and walk for two. That would help my performance a tiny bit! After passing the 39k waypoint I rarely glanced at my stopwatch. And when I did it was just to reassure myself that, barring any major disaster, I would finish on time. My legs were painful, but I had no cramp. My shoes were a bit tight, but that was nothing more than a slight irritation. Looking for the positives at all times I reminded myself that I no longer had to do any mental arithmetic. I just had to yomp! I had to keep on keeping on!

There was a good one kilometre of the route going north east up *Quai Wilson* towards the U turn at *Parc Mon Repos*, and another one kilometre going back down again. As I went north I could clearly see the runners ahead of me coming south. A fair few of them. After the U turn I had my best unobstructed view of the runners behind me. There were a good number of them as well. I was nowhere near last.

I was catching up with some of the runners ahead of me. Walkers to be honest, not runners at this final stage. I was yomping, they were walking, I was constantly passing them, one by one, and I could see more coming into view ahead of me all the time. Unlike a lot of the lonelier stretches earlier that day, this final kilometre, in this final ten minutes before the sweeper bus, put me in proximity with two or three dozen entrants. All of them resigned to walking to the finishing line, all mindful of the mythical sweeper bus just behind us. By all accounts as we went south on *Quai Wilson* we ought to have seen the sweeper bus going north. It wasn't there.

What really puzzled me was that I was now in the midst of so many runners, when generally I had been relatively isolated from runners for the past couple of hours. Anyway, the debate now was how I was going to handle the last few hundred metres.

My habit is to run the last stretch, partly to please the crowds, and partly to satisfy my own ego. And to run it with the utmost care, checking exactly where I place my feet, avoiding manhole covers, drain covers, and any defects in the road. No sprinting, just a meaningful slow running pace. I wanted no mishaps at this critical stage of the race. The question was whether I would run for 500, or 400 or 300m at the end. I was unsure about maintaining a running pace for 500m and so I chose to play it safe, to run the final 300m.

The *Hotel de la Paix* came into view. By my estimation that left me with 400m of the course. With my "run the final 300m" mentality firmly set in my brain I estimated that the right moment to switch would be when I turned left off *Quai du Mont Blanc* and onto the bridge itself. Reaching the apex of the sweeping 90° left turn would be the trigger. I would transition from walking to running for the last time in this race. Before reaching the turn I glanced towards the finish line, looking for the photographers, I wanted to have this finish recorded for posterity. That hadn't happened on my first marathon because by the time I reached the finish all the photographers had gone home!

As I reached the apex of the bend I stepped up the pace, the walk became a run. And at that precise moment one of the spectators (who had clearly clocked my name and the UK flag on my bib) shouted in his brash North American accent "come on Paul, you can do it"!

And I knew I could. And I was still grateful for the vote of confidence.

And I ran. I checked my stopwatch. It said 5 hrs 51 mins 40 secs. I could now see the clock above the finish line, and that said 5 hrs 54 mins 57 secs. Even according to the "race timing" I was going to finish in less than six hours.

Now get ready for the official photo! Look calm, look relaxed, look totally in control. I spotted the photographer to the left and in front of the finish line, and as I approached I smiled, looked directly at the lens, gave him a thumbs up sign, and internally I allowed myself a silent scream of joy. Placing my foot on the sensor I crossed the line in 5 hrs 52 mins 31 secs.

That was a fabulous experience, I had been in control throughout, I had run better and for longer than last time, I had managed the unexpectedly intense levels of pain, and I had at no time stopped moving due to fatigue. My only physical stops had been at 3k to remove my top, and at about 17k to help the British Indian girl sort out the photo. I looked for Mr Japan, but I hadn't seen him going north as I was coming south on *Quai Wilson*. By now I was sure that he would miss the cut off, and in any case I assumed that he had probably retired due to injury. Nor had I seen Mr Stocky from Manchester. As far back as the 15k point I guessed that *he* had already reasoned that he was unprepared for this sort of distance. I assumed that he had also retired.

With my finishers medal and a bottle of water I watched some others cross the finish line, for just one or two minutes more. I had intended to see the young husband and wife (the ones with the stopwatch mix up) make it to the end. However, my legs hurt like mad, my shoes were pinching my feet, and my shirt was wetter than I had ever known it before. I wanted dry socks, dry shoes and the full change of clothes from my drop bag. I found the correct truck, picked up my bag from the few dozen that remained (nobody checked my bib number against the tag on my bag) and I crossed the street to a shop front with a recessed doorway where I changed. I had never before had such a buzz from putting on clean socks and fresh shoes! I parked that thought in my brain as well. Remember, a change of shoes even if it's a perfectly sunny day! During my race I had so many mental notes which I needed to write down. So much information to contribute towards my third marathon.

As I sat in that shop doorway I was both elated and dejected, again. The same as last time! Elated that I had completed my second marathon, I had beaten the cut off time, and that automatically meant that I had a new personal best. Dejected, because I had wanted to do it in five hours not six, and inexplicably I had encountered a lot more pain than on any of my previous long runs.

Did I really want to do a third marathon? Five years later? Aged 60?

The thought going through my head was "my distance is 10k and I should just stick to doing that".

Chapter 10 - Third Time Lucky and Unlucky

Mixed Emotions

I really hadn't understood why I'd had so much muscle fatigue during the Geneva Marathon, and why I needed to slow down at the 25k waypoint. Clearly the pattern was similar to marathon one in Milton Keynes. I was delighted to have finished, comfortably ahead of the sweeper bus, and with a new personal best. To be honest, it's not too hard to beat 6 hours 28, nor is the time of 5 hours 52 especially impressive.

The conscientious marathon training had started two years earlier with me trying to incrementally improve my stamina and distance. I knew the Geneva route reasonably well, because had done the half marathon the year before and had cycled the full course a few days before the event. By 2018 I was also a much more experienced runner. Well equipped, with my own water supply, no energy gel, boiled sweets if needed, and my clothing was precisely what I wanted and what I felt comfortable wearing. The preparation had been done thoroughly.

However, I was disappointed that I couldn't figure out what had truly gone wrong at the 20k - 25k stage in each marathon. I didn't remember having muscle fatigue that badly when I had done long training runs.

Resting at home that evening I focussed on the good points. The achievement, the time, the medal, the quality of the course, the absence of flooding, the waypoints (clear, accurate and in kilometres), the water stations, the spectators everywhere, and especially the crowds in the city centre. The crowds on the final kilometre were cheering on every single runner. My second marathon had exactly the right atmosphere, whereas my first had very little atmosphere indeed. I went to bed, legs still feeling sore, though nothing prevented me from sleeping really well that night. When I woke up the next morning, the pain was less intense but it was still there. I went to the bathroom, inspected my calves in the mirror, and the problem was obvious. I had sunburn! All the way from the where my shorts stopped to where my socks started. It wasn't muscle fatigue.

Not only that, I had made it worse by slowing down and staying out in the sun longer. Mid race I had mistakenly diagnosed muscle fatigue, when in fact I had failed to apply sun cream to the back of my legs, and had caught a bit too much sun on an extremely hot day. By slowing down I had subjected myself to more sun over a longer period, and not only that, the sun during the later part of the day is more intense when it's higher in the sky. Well! I won't make that mistake again!

And I had nobody to blame but myself.

Right! That's it then! I'm going to have to do another one! I'm going to have to do a third marathon and prove to myself that I'm not stupid! And this time I going to do it properly!

It's probably true:

"you spend your first two marathons learning how *not* to run a marathon"

60 Year Old Paul

When I was 55 years old I had already been toying with the idea of doing one marathon every year in order to maintain my health and fitness, and especially my weight control. I had pencilled in Milton Keynes for May 2019, one year after the Geneva Marathon.

By this time in 2018, I could run 10k at the drop of a hat. That wasn't the case back in 2005 and 2006 when my first 10k had led to profound feelings of dread, and fear of the unknown.

I could do 21k too, without much trouble. Hence, if I could regularly run 42k without hesitation or fear, the way that I can do the lesser distances, then surely my next marathon would be a push over?

After all, some people do ultra marathons, ridiculous distances, so it must be feasible to build up the stamina to do "a mere 42k" with few worries. I have to make 42k normal, the way that 10k is normal now.

Yes! Dream on!

Getting Serious

I mapped out a training plan, intending to do some long distance work on a regular basis, and to maintain a limited program of entering official races.

That summer of 2018 I went to Wexford and Dublin, and did 10k training runs in both. I went to a Tech Conference in Birmingham in October 2018 and took time off on the Sunday morning to run the official Birmingham Half Marathon.

It rained! And that gave me my best official time over 21k, a time of 2 hrs 7 mins 51 secs. It also taught me that a wet iPhone 6 will not work after hours in the rain, and so I was unable to phone my wife at the end and tell her I'd finished! Since then, my phone sits inside a small plastic zip lock bag in the pocket in the backpack.

Getting Very Serious

Allied to my new found passion for being serious, I decided that I needed perfectly accurate measurements for my training runs. Road layouts in central London change sometimes. Building sites appear, footpaths close, and the arrival of the Thames Tideway works at Blackfriars had a devasting impact on one of my preferred training routes. I was convinced that some of my runs had become longer, as I had been forced to use different roads in order to cover roughly the same routes. And I was not convinced that Google maps was giving me accurate fine detail for "walking" routes.

I bought a measuring wheel.

That meant that I walked and walked and walked considerable distances, all over central London, pushing this wheel ahead of me. With pen and paper at hand, I would stop every kilometre to make notes. For the first time I knew exactly where my periodic way points were located. I also learnt that my 10k route was actually 10.26k. Should I modify my route to make it exactly 10k? No! My 7k route is actually 6.876k. Over the years, my log had times and distances for all these routes and I didn't want to adjust the history. Or to modify things for the future, because I wanted to continue comparing like with like. I still run the same 10k route, covering 10.26k and record the time in my log.

I used the measuring wheel so much that it eventually broke. By that time it had proved its worth and I have a lovely set of route maps. I couldn't do that with the odometer on the bike, because a lot of my London routes are pedestrian only, and I'm not the sort of rule breaker who would cycle that far on footpaths.

The Injury Puzzle

One week after the Birmingham Half Marathon (October 2018) I was out at 6.00am in the morning, in the dark, and I suffered my first troubling injury. A raised manhole cover outside the National Theatre on the South Bank tripped me up.

The stumble almost had me on the ground, but I managed to prevent that by jarring my left leg. Although I prevented a fall, I had felt the force of the impact travel up my left leg, and do something to my hip. I recovered my composure, I ran a further 50 metres and then stopped! I had done 4k of my 10k run.

I've stumbled in the past, occasionally I've pulled a muscle. Sometimes I resume my run, and sometimes I choose to walk home. This one was different. Very uncomfortable. I tried walking a bit. I wasn't going to be able to walk the remaining 6k.

Slowly, I crossed over Waterloo Bridge in order to take a train home from Temple. I did no mid week runs for 7 days after that, because my hip felt just a little weird. But I did go out on the following Sunday intending to stick to my program, and to cover 25k that day.

That would have kept me in line with my training plan leading towards the Milton Keynes Marathon in May 2019. It didn't work out like that! I had set out later than usual that morning, I managed 21k in 2 hrs 15 mins, and then I stopped. Partly due to fatigue, and partly due to the sheer numbers of people who were out in Battersea Park on a Sunday morning. I really don't like having to negotiate footpaths when they begin to get crowded. The minor niggle with the left hip was not really the issue, though it probably played a part. As I walked the final 4k home I constantly thought about the stumble at the National Theatre. Had it caused distress to the bone or the joint, or was it a soft tissue injury?

I decided to manage the injury myself, principally because the NHS had not been that helpful in 2012 when I had RSI. I decided to take time off from running and do a lot of walking instead. That also meant that my idea of doing marathons every year was shelved, and that Milton Keynes in 2019 was no longer viable.

Returning to an earlier plan, I promised myself that I would still follow a five year pattern and do my third marathon when I turned 60. Plenty of time to get ready for that, and plenty of time to manage the hip injury I thought. Or to seek medical advice if it really was a bone injury, and not soft tissue. I put it down to "greater trochanteric bursitis". It would vanish for a while, months even, and then return. It remained truly trivial for ages, though I still had lingering doubts about my own self diagnosis skills.

My notes from my log on 29 Apr 2020 say "bursitis has returned - two weeks now - getting worse - really annoying - especially when I try to go to sleep - taking ibuprofen and doing ITB stretches". What I wanted to know was, was it soft tissue, or was it a bone problem? Eventually (shunning my own NHS GP) I paid to see a private GP on 10 Nov 2020. He wrangled my left leg in all manner of contortions, and declared that I was fine. If you had any bone or joint issues, that would have hurt!

Iliotibial Band Syndrome
www.wikipedia.org

My online medical sleuthing continued. I established from serious websites that I did have iliotibial band syndrome. The QR code for Wikipedia is given so that you can get a simple overview. I experienced the pain at the top of the femur (the greater trochanter) rather than at the bottom. It was a regular thing for years. On and off for weeks at a time, and it finally vanished after I lost significant weight in 2023. I finally learnt a sure fire way to lose weight and keep it off. Running involves one type of system. Weight management requires a different system. Nowadays, I don't have half of the injury problems I used to have.

However, on account of old age, the few injuries I do have tend to stick around for longer.

The Great North Run

I raced against Sir Mo Farah in The Great North Run in 2019. And I let him win! The Great North Run is the world's biggest *half marathon*. So I thought it would be interesting to do it at least once.

On the Saturday, one day before the race, I checked the route by car. I couldn't cycle it this time, because the start is on a motorway. On the Sunday I joined the pen marked 2 hours 30, amongst 56,000 entrants, all spread out along part of the inner city motorway in Newcastle.

The start was the worst experience I've ever had at an official race. It should be renamed The Great North Apology. Too many people, all bumping into each other! "Sorry!" "Sorry!" "Sorry!" It wasn't until about Mile 3 that I found just a little personal space and could start running properly. Though I was still brutally confined by everyone around me.

The water stations were the biggest shock. Although I was content with my own backpack and water supply, my rhythm was unavoidably disrupted by thousands of runners at each water station. Instead of using lightweight disposable cups (which I had seen at every single official race in the past) The Great North Run had small plastic bottles. Runners picked one up, unscrewed the cap, dropped the cap on the floor, drank what they wanted and then chucked the half full plastic bottle roughly in the direction of the bins a few metres further along. Being generous, I might assume that half of the field was ahead of me, of which half of them wanted bottled water. That meant that 14,000 bottle tops lay ahead of me. You never see that on TV!

It wasn't as bad as treading on Lego bricks. But it was awful trying to run through a minefield of hundreds of hard blue plastic bottle tops strewn across the road everywhere, and then having to navigate a "ball pit" of small plastic bottles which had never made it to the side of the road.

As I passed the water station at Mile 8 I'd had enough. I started walking. Carefully I picked my way through this latest minefield of plastic, and then I just continued walking. I may have jogged a little in a few places, but I was not having a good day. If it wasn't plastic getting in the way, it was half empty sachets of energy gel. That shocked me too, that runners would discard gel in the middle of the road, and not at the side. These things stick to the soles of your shoes, and if the plastic packet soon disappears, the tacky gel stays there for longer, letting you know that it's trying to glue every one of your footsteps to the road. Owing to the mass of people it was impossible to see the road ahead clearly and to avoid any of this mess.

Physically, I was absolutely fine. Mentally, I was deeply troubled that anybody could stage an event this way, and that so many runners had a total disregard for their fellow runners. I finished in 2 hrs 57 mins 56 secs. My slowest half marathon ever.

Crowd management at the end is both good and bad. We had to hastily rearrange our rendezvous on account of closed roads and pedestrian one way systems. Though eventually I found my family, and inching forwards, it took us 1 hour 20 minutes to queue for a train at South Shields station.

Never again.

Soon after The Great North Run, right at the end of September 2019, I was out on one of my regular early morning runs, at about 5.30am when it was still dark and I hit a loose paving stone badly. I hadn't seen the problem.

That was it! Decision made!

Halfway through the 10k training run I started walking home and I warned myself that I should not run when it was dark. The street lighting along The Thames Path was not helping me spot danger signals.

During the winter of 2019/20 I did a mix of running and walking. I bought a cross trainer for use at home, as there is a lesser risk of impact injuries from running. The bursitis flared up again, and my enthusiasm for a third marathon waned. In general, injuries were becoming more common than when I was younger. And life suddenly became more complicated.

The Covid 19 pandemic struck. My son was not enjoying his first year at Uni, because all his lectures and tutorials had moved on line. Some of my customers went out of business, hence the pandemic also affected my business. It wasn't life threatening amounts of money, but my income went down by about 20%.

A short time later, and completely unrelated to the Covid 19 pandemic, my father died, and then my father in law died. Both within a few weeks of each other.

This bizarre, and exhausting set of circumstances pushed the idea of a third marathon right to the back of my mind.

I would soon be 60 years old. My original pattern of one marathon every five years was embedded in my mind. However, I reasoned that I was answerable to nobody, and that a delay of one more year, or two, would be fine.

To be honest, I didn't have to do *a third marathon* at all.

Discovering a sure fire method of losing weight, in June 2023 (see the next chapter), made all the difference. In the space of four days my BMI went down from 29.6 to 28.9, a reduction of 2.27%. It was astonishing. It also rekindled my enthusiasm for all things health and fitness related. It was summer, the days were longer, and there would be no running in the dark. I could now run as much as I liked.

I started looking for marathon dates in early 2024. I would be 61 years old by then, but that's OK. It's my agenda, I can change it if I want to. I took it easy through July and August 2023. No races booked, no strict running agenda, just a pleasant resumption of regular running, mainly over shorter distances. I was simply happy to be back in the right frame of mind, constantly improving my weight loss campaign and improving my running campaign at the same time.

Then step forward one younger brother! And say "I have entered the Tonbridge Half Marathon on 1 Oct 2023". Brilliant! I didn't have a marathon date in mind yet, but I was accustomed to my system of doing some serious running as I prepare. So I registered for the Tonbridge Half Marathon. I would basically have the whole of September to get ready, running in London and in Fukuoka.

Looking ahead to 2024 I shortlisted the marathons in Peterborough and Boston as potential targets. Boston, Lincs, had a particular appeal as it was billed as "the flattest marathon in the UK" with excellent scope for getting a personal best.

My 2024 marathon programme was germinating, but the only thing that was truly certain was that I was doing the Tonbridge Half Marathon on 1 Oct 2023. That was a little sooner than I might otherwise have chosen as I hadn't yet fleshed out a plan. In any case, I'd done many 10k runs, and a lot of 21k runs, so I wasn't particularly fazed by entering an official *half marathon* which was just five weeks away. I trained diligently during those five weeks, increasing my distances and improving my stamina.

Three days to go, Thursday 28 Sep 2023, I set off on a regular 10k training run at about 6.40am. It was twilight, just before sunrise at 6.56am. Everything was normal until fractionally before my 4k waypoint. My left knee hurt. Badly! Really badly. No idea why. Should I stop? Should I run on? The sun was up, normal daylight, and I hadn't seen any problems. However, I lasted barely another 10 or 20 metres before I stopped. The knee was hurting much more than it had ever done before. And I was three days away from the Tonbridge Half which was now a firm part of my training for my third marathon.

What should I do? I sat down. There were some park benches right there, between Gabriels Wharf and the Oxo Tower. Normally I never sit down, not even when I pull a muscle. I was truly puzzled. I've done that path hundreds of times before without incident. I sat down to debate my next move.

It's OK to not be OK. I walked home.

At the local pharmacy that morning I bought a size D TubiGrip (an elasticated, cylindrical bandage) and wore it all day at the office. The next morning I went back and bought one size bigger. The knee had no swelling, but I started taking anti inflammatories as a precaution.

I deferred my own decision about withdrawing, until the Sunday morning of the race. My body clock woke me up at 4.52am just before my 5.00am alarm. This is normal for me! On with the TubiGrip. Walk around the flat a bit. Minutes later, outside, walk roughly 100m, so far so good, turn around and run the 100m back home. Yes, OK. Clearly not perfect, but I'm OK for a gentle run. The sensation in the knee is not really "pain" just a little bit of "discomfort".

In Tonbridge, I met my brother, explained my new "gentle" strategy, and said that my revised pace (with a pace sheet on my right wrist) would get me to the finish in 2 hrs 37 mins. Any time would be OK as long as I beat the 3 hour cut off. He was on for something like 1 hr 45 mins and achieved that.

Wearing a TubiGrip for the first time on a race, I tried to run strictly to my pace sheet. My home made pace sheet for the race was in miles, not my familiar kilometres. It sort of worked out, although the ups and downs of The South Downs led me slow down for a couple of sections. I finished in 2 hrs 38 mins 32 secs. To be honest, I was delighted with that. I had nursed a knee injury, and had safely completed the race.

I was 60 years old when I did that race. Over the years I have seen many runners, some far younger than me, wearing knee supports. I've never needed one before. I intended to wear mine for a few weeks until I felt that things were back to normal. I scaled back my distance, and in spite of some very feeble whinging, the knee was coping fine. Until day 15 of the TubiGrip. Then it said "enough". I knew that I had to address a proper remedy. Proper rest!

Swimming! The other exercise I do is swimming, but I do it very rarely. And interestingly I'd never been to the Olympic pool in Stratford. I resolved to rest my knee completely for six weeks and to swim one mile every Sunday. I was 10 years old when I first completed 64 lengths of a 25m pool. One mile. I've done it many times.

On six consecutive Sundays in October and November 2023 I went to the Olympic pool to do 32 lengths of 50m. The knee twinged a few times during the swims, but there was nothing alarming. Walking was fine too. A trial 5k run on 30 Nov 2023 told me that the recovery period had been well worth it. I was ready to resume my marathon training programme, and I was just about on track to complete a marathon in the following spring.

Boston or Peterborough

I weighed up the pros and cons of running either the Peterborough or the Boston Marathons. The races are similar, and either would have been fine, though the date was the deciding factor. In early December I registered for the 28 Apr 2024 Boston Marathon, paid £35.00 and stated that my expected time was 5 hrs 30.

Slow Down The Pace Paul

My pace sheet became increasingly important. When you have the habit of starting too fast you need a rethink. What exactly are you trying to do? I'm trying to live a long, fit and healthy life. I am not competing with anybody else. Having put the recent knee trouble behind me, I started aiming for "mundane" times. Mundane to everybody except me. My pace sheet said run 10k in 72 minutes, and I was still doing them in about 67 minutes. I forced myself to adopt a "grandad pace" and I learnt to go slower. The pace I wanted to maintain for a whole marathon was 7 minutes 39 per kilometre.

I had just about mastered the "grandad pace" and then the old injury returned. I mean the really old one, the one that I had completely forgotten about. The one from 1983 when I was 20 years old.

The Mysterious Case of the Bone That Didn't Break

What the RSI debacle in 2012 had taught me is that if you have multiple pain points, then the one that screams the loudest masks the pain from the other ones. In 2023 my left knee had four pain points and each one was different. In the early days I hadn't really thought about multiple pain points. It became obvious later on!

So I spent lots of time online researching knee problems. Studying anatomy. On the discussion boards of running websites the most common complaint seemed to be "the knee" in general and it was hard to get down to specifics. I wanted to understand the science. I read about "shallow grooves" in which the patella slipped around, and about Patellofemoral Pain Syndrome.

My left *patella* didn't feel the same as the right one, but perhaps that was my inexpert hand just detecting that the left *knee* in general didn't feel the same as the right knee. I started making accurate notes about where each pain occurred.

Yes, sometimes it was the patella, the lower centre of the patella, or at least that's what it felt like. Sometimes it was the head of the fibula (left hand side of my left knee), and sometimes it was the medial condyle of the tibia (right hand side of my left knee). And then sometimes it was a few centimetres lower down the fibula, over to the left. A few centimetres lower down the left fibula, over to the left?

That was where I had a stress fracture when I was 20 years old. It was caused by a hefty jump where I landed hard on both feet, though clearly the left leg had taken more of the impact.

In 1983 the shock from the landing was transmitted upwards, leading to a minor stress fracture, at the top of the shaft, just below the neck of the fibula. I didn't even know this at the time. I thought it was trivial, and I simply took it easy for a while to let the pain subside. I remember it happening, it was on my way to a football field, and due the injury I decided to sit out the game.

Some Medical Science

Dr Jānis Šavlovskis (radiologist) and Kristaps Raits (digital 3D artist) have some excellent illustrations at www.anatomystandard.com

www.anatomystandard.com

"In a practical sense, the fibula does not carry any significant weight of the body. The function of the fibula is limited by muscles, and by the attached ligaments coming from the knee and the ankle. Surgical intervention of the mid third of the fibula does not cause a significant biomechanical disturbance."

"And due to the limited functional load on the bone, a fracture of the shaft of the fibula, under some circumstances, may remain undiscovered."

There you have it! The expert website says "may remain undiscovered". That was me in 1983. I didn't even know about the fracture until I had an x-ray done one year later. And I didn't learn the science until 40 years later in 2023.

In 1984 (a full one year after the impact) the stress fracture had opened up again. And it was much more painful the second time around! Then (aged 21) I had it x-rayed and the doctor helped me drill down through the history. There was a very clear trace of a bone callus where the stress fracture at the top of the shaft of the fibula had healed, and the x-ray showed that this fracture had reopened.

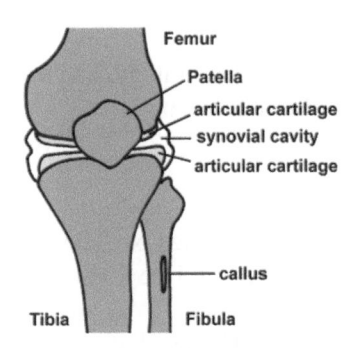

Left knee - anterior view - not to scale

At least in 1984 I now knew what had happened in 1983. And then I forgot about it again. Until the cold weather arrived in late November 2023 and the bone ached in exactly the same place and in exactly the same way. I was pretty sure that the old stress fracture was playing up again. Probably the tiniest hint of a disturbance to the healed callus or to the fracture beneath it. I could feel it in my bones!

Then again, I probably had multiple small injuries in and around the knee, all of which piped up from time to time shouting "me, me, me" before calming down once more to let some other patch of distress have its turn. Multiple pain points, multiple defects, all conspiring to act in concert and play a mischievous game of hide and seek with me.

I also learnt that (whether we're runners or not) joints get worse as we get older, and that synovial fluid, not blood, is how the body maintains and repairs damage to the articular cartilage cushioning the bones at your joints. There are no blood vessels in the deepest part of our joints. So, instead of healthy blood cells doing the repair job with various nutrients, synovial fluid does it by utilising hyaluronic acid. And unfortunately we humans do not produce an abundance of hyaluronic acid, and older humans seem to produce even less of it.

Although I'm generally not in favour of health supplements (I prefer a diet of good fresh food) I decided to buy both hyaluronic acid and calcium supplements in order to accelerate the healing process. Hyaluronic acid to work on the cartilage, and calcium to repair the stress fracture. Whether they worked or not is hard to say, because I would need to compare me to a clone of me, one who used the supplements, and one who didn't.

What I did learn was that I had to take it easy for a while. I was already on track with my gentle recovery, and I was planning a newer, more cautious approach to marathon running.

Armed with my new "grandad pace" strategy, and my new medical knowledge, I was ready to be a model of pragmatism.

Disaster Strikes Again

Maybe I should give up running past the Oxo Tower, because that's where it all went wrong again, on Boxing Day, 26 Dec 2023.

When you run westwards on the Thames Path past Sea Containers House you approach the Oxo Tower, and you have two options. To run alongside the wall by the river, onto the narrow, uncovered footpath with the abrupt 90° turns at the other end, or you can run on the wider, covered footpath with a gentle slalom past all the shops, and avoid the two 90° pinch points at the end. I habitually use the wider one because sharp 90° turns are not my thing.

On Boxing Day, as I passed the threshold into the covered walkway my left knee howled in pain. For heaven's sake why? Why now? After all the care, and research, and revision to the plans, and after donkeys years of running that exact same route, why did my knee give up precisely there? There aren't even any sunken drains or raised manhole covers, just a gentle slope from uncovered to covered walkway.

Have you ever walked up or down a set of steps, anticipating the final step, only to discover that there's one more step beyond that?

Your foot moves differently, especially if you were going down the steps, and your leg just about copes with the unexpected additional drop, and you steady yourself, thinking "oh, there was one more step". That's what had happened to me at the Oxo Tower. My foot went down a little more than I expected. Finally it struck the ground, transmitted the impact up my leg, and my left knee howled.

I was only able to work all that out when I went back to inspect the troublesome location a few days later. The slope is not a perfectly uniform slope. Nor is it a step. It's one slope with a combination of three separate gradients, all of which normally present no problem. I had been along there hundreds of times. Though this time the length of my stride, the miniscule difference in the gradients, and the already weak knee all combined to end my training run on the spot.

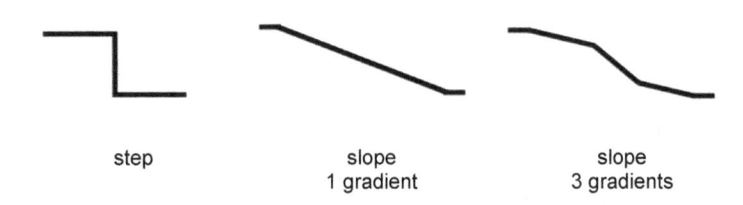

step   slope
1 gradient   slope
3 gradients

illustration only - not to scale

The stumble was so bad, and the walking so troublesome, that I hobbled only 400m before detouring to the nearest bus stop to get me home. Bus routes in central London operate a limited service on Boxing Day. Thankfully!

Deferment

With this latest recurrence, I had no option but to defer my Boston Marathon entry from April 2024 to April 2025. More importantly, instead of giving myself six weeks off for recovery (as I had done the previous time) I allowed myself an open ended recovery period.

In spite of that, I was still impatient to get a third marathon done before I turned 62, so I started looking for more options for later in the year. There was the Loch Ness Marathon on 28 Sep 2024 and the Chelmsford Marathon on 13 Oct 2024.

Loch Ness, appealed to me. A scenic *point to point* race covering 42k in roughly a straight line. Departing from Inverness, they take you to the start line by bus, and you run back. Chelmsford is a much smaller event, covering small country roads from Central Park to Willingale (the long way around) and back again. I registered for Loch Ness and booked hotels for seven nights away from London. Both the entry fee and the hotels were pricey, but I like Scotland!

In the early part of 2024 it occurred to me that the Highlands can sometimes be wet. What would I do if it rained during the race? I didn't want to repeat the Wokingham Half Marathon strategy of wearing a kagool. The idea took root was that I would wear a thin plastic pac-a-mac, over my dayglo jacket, over my T shirt. The sort of cheap, flimsy pac-a-mac that you see tourists wearing on open top double decker bus tours.

I waited for a rainy day in London to test out my theory. It took time for that day to arrive, but it was bound to arrive sooner or later, and it coincided with a day for one of my slow 10k runs. And it was proper rain, but not too heavy. I put on the pac-a-mac, and set off running in what turned out to be my own personal transportable sauna outfit. I was hot by the 2k waypoint, too hot. I stopped at 4k and removed the plastic mac. I completed the 10k in the rain, my dayglo jacket was wet through by the end. The baseball cap kept most of the rain off my glasses, and the exertion of running (albeit slowly) was more than enough to keep me warm in spite of the rain.

So I decided that when I do the Loch Ness Marathon I will carry a pac-a-mac just in case. I will wear it only if there is absolutely torrential rain. As Billy Connolly says of Scotland:

> *"There's no such thing as bad weather - only inappropriate clothing."*

Sporting my unbreakable spirit, if it's a day full of ordinary rain I will be running in my dayglo jacket, T shirt and shorts. And I will get wet. And I will salute my willpower.

Health is Threat Management

Months and months passed. January to August 2024 were a real mixed bag of emotion and ability, injury and demi-fitness. I went to Japan in February and I could only walk my running routes. I was back there in May by which time I was running again. The Boston and Peterborough Marathons, came and went without me. My entire training program was in disarray. There was a bit of running and a lot of walking. In June I was back to only walking. Trying out 5k, then 10k, then 20k. By this time, I normally wore the TubiGrip when, and only when, I was doing exercise

One day in mid June I walked my London Six Bridges half marathon route and I stopped at 16k due to my knee complaining. I had a late breakfast at Embankment Gardens Café, and after a 45 minute break, I resumed the walk completing the remaining 5k at a distinctly geriatric pace.

I scaled back my exercise to a handful of timed 5k walks each week. My fitness gradually improved. One day, completely by mistake, I forgot to wear the TubiGrip on my left knee. I didn't notice it was missing until about the 2k waypoint. Actually, it was no longer needed. I was fine. I didn't wear it again. Six weeks passed. Lots of walking, but six weeks devoid of any running.

On 28 Jul 2024 I set out to walk my 21k route again. This time I wanted to power walk it in less than 3 hours, to see if I could "walk the Loch Ness Marathon" in less than 6 hours. By the 3k waypoint I knew that my walking pace was inadequate, so even though I was dressed in everyday clothes, sporting my ordinary everyday Reebok trainers, I started running. I yomped my half marathon route! Repeatedly walking 3k then running 1k, inhibited by my wallet and the iPhone in my pocket, though aided by a bum bag which contained small disposable water pouches.

That 21k training "run" took me 2hrs 48mins 58secs, faster than I had achieved on the 2019 Great North Run. More importantly, there was no pain. My knee was as near normal as I could imagine. In all it had taken more than 6 months of cautious recovery, and I felt as if I could do a marathon and beat 6 hours. Loch Ness was on!

Canguilhem had taught me to manage the threats. My running during the hours of darkness had ended, my routes had changed to avoid the accident black spots, and my recovery periods had lengthened in order to allow damaged tissue to fully recover. I had adapted to my environment. An environment which included the changing characteristics and geography of London (changes to my preferred running routes), and the changing attributes of an old man who was slowly discovering what it's like to become very gradually, and very slightly infirm.

I ran my London Six Bridges half marathon route the following Sunday, in 2 hrs 33 mins 15 secs, and as I finished I had a massive dopamine rush. After months of nursing injuries I was normal, I was finally fit again. I had just run for two and half hours with no rests and no walking! I returned to my standard training programme. Two midweek 10k runs, and a longer run on Sundays, immediately incrementing the Sunday distance to 25k, three weeks of that, then two at 30k, and a further two at 35k.

I was cutting it fine, but I was on track, and I set my sights on Loch Ness.

By Tuesday 6 Aug 2024 I was back to being my normal self, following my normal routine. I had a lovely gentle 10k run, trying to mimic my ideal marathon pace, 7 minute 39 kilometres. I found it really difficult to go that slow. However, at about the 3k waypoint, I had an epiphany. I had discovered the secret sauce. It's not speed, it's not distance, it's all about endurance! Actually, I said that in 2011. You might remember in Chapter 4 that my task included "work on endurance".

I had forgotten that basic principle, and for years my mind had been focussed on managing to run further and further. What I really needed to focus on was running for longer and longer. Running for literally hours on end. Duration! Not distance! If I could maintain an unbroken slow run for 5 hours and 30 minutes, then it would automatically follow that I would have completed 42k.

I was at home that evening, and had a stupid, trivial accident which resulted in a broken toe on my left foot! Maybe it was just sprained, but it was bent. Seven weeks before the Loch Ness Marathon! Nine weeks before Chelmsford!

First the left hip, then the left knee, and now my left foot!

That same evening, Tuesday 6 Aug 2024, I had been working on a draft of this chapter, and before injuring myself I had just written:

I needed to fixate on a constant running pace, even a slow one, and just stick to it for hours and hours. I had found the secret sauce. I had less than eight weeks to go before Loch Ness. Could I turn my new found discovery into my new found policy, and stick to it? No more yomping when I'm fatigued. Consistency and persistency! Run slower! From the outset!"

Parts of this chapter ended up with a drastic rewrite! In any case, having a broken toe meant another recovery break, and it meant that the 29 Sep 2024 Loch Ness Marathon was off. I withdrew. Third time lucky and unlucky, and unlucky again and again!

Six weeks' rest was needed. And then possibly three to four weeks of training after that? Oh boy, I was cutting it fine! Could I finish my marathon prep in time for Chelmsford on 13 Oct 2024?

If I wasn't fit for the Chelmsford Marathon then I would have to wait for Boston to come around again. A further six month wait for April 2025.

Let's return to my comment above about the *secret sauce*. It had germinated when I was doing some research on fatigue and *hitting the wall*.

Hitting the Wall

A book on marathon running wouldn't be complete if it didn't mention this phenomenon. Was I ever at risk of *hitting the wall*?

Short answer, no! Not in the classic, catastrophic sense!

Given that I've been carrying excess weight for most of my running career, and I was slow, I thought that there was little risk that I would use up all of the available energy resources which my body could muster.

"Hitting the wall" or "the bonk" is used to describe a complete and instant loss of energy after the body has used all of the available glycogen stores, pulling every last resource from the muscles themselves and from the liver. Runners simply collapse as their legs will carry them no further.

It's avoided by carb loading in advance of the run, and by taking on food or drink containing carbohydrates during the run. Reducing the intensity of the run reduces the likelihood of "hitting the wall".

My few involuntary changes from running to walking have probably been the body's inbuilt mechanism overruling my brain, and thus preventing a total collapse.

A change of tempo (a complete stop or a lesser effort) gives the body time to work its fatty acids and release more energy. Apparently, ten minutes is normally enough to respond to increased demands.

My broken toe was not as troubling as the broken finger which I had suffered in the past. It was strapped up neatly to its neighbour. Although my running had stopped, everything else in life carried on as normal.

On the bank holiday Monday on 26 Aug 2024 I went to Chelmsford by train, and I cycled the marathon route. Oh dear! Not good! There's an entire blogpost about it!

Chelmsford Recce
www.dontreadmyblog.com

Having had first hand experience of the course, I decided to register anyway. I resumed my training on 19 Sep 2024 with a gentle 7k run. I had only 24 days left to make up for lost time. But I now had the secret sauce! Would I be ready for Chelmsford? Did I have enough time to do some long slow runs? Would I actually do the race?

I was in a similar position to the year before. In 2023 I had waited until the morning of the race to make a decision about the Tonbridge Half Marathon.

This time, on the morning of the Chelmsford Marathon 2024, I could simply choose not to take the train there.

Or I could get on the 0726 from Liverpool Street Station.

Chapter 11 - Weight Management and Calories

King's College London

King's College London is one of the eighteen constituent colleges of the University of London. It's where I did my teacher training during 1999-2000. Naturally, after I graduated I joined the Alumni Association and have been along to some of their activities. Occasionally these events produce an absolute gem, and one of those happened on 14 Jun 2023, the inaugural King's Impact Reception.

Six faculties across the University were represented. It was a pleasant evening with demonstrations of various cutting edge technologies, and with talks and presentations about new innovations from the medical school and the business school. I have never been in a room so full of intelligent people all doing good! Seasoned conference-goers will know, that away from the main event, some of the golden nuggets of the day can often be found in the informal discussions in the "hallway track". The unplanned encounters and conversations that take place in the corridors between the main sessions.

I love the "hallway track"! And this one, at this event, produced the best gem of all. I was chatting with Professor Richard Trembath (Health & Life Sciences) about nutrition, when our discussion naturally turned to Fish & Chips. It's on my blog if you want the full picture.

Fish & Chips
www.dontreadmyblog.com

To cut a long story short, that conversation kick-started a serious effort on my part to understand a bit more about nutrition and calories. Such was the impact that for the first time in my life I prepared a detailed food diary which actually included counting the calories. I did that for three weeks. My running log has a "weight" column and I can tell you that in that three week period I lost 2.5kg. That was astonishing.

So that's how people do it, they actually count the calories, and they lose weight!

> **Warning**
>
> This system might seem a bit drastic, and a bit like hard work. That's why people *don't* follow it. It takes some effort, and a bit of commitment, and it does work. I challenge you to do calorie counting for seven days in a row. It works, believe me! It's worth reading this whole chapter to understand how it's done.
>
> Weigh yourself at the start and the end.
>
> Log everything you eat and the calorie count. If you're conscientious you'll change your eating habits and you will see how calorie counting leads to weight loss. In my case my snacking on sandwiches, on chocolate, and on cereal stopped completely. My consumption of apples went up massively. Household expenditure on snacks has practically vanished, and the money we spend on apples is three times higher than before.
>
> If that's the price I have to pay for a successful weight loss system then I'm willing to pay it. Don't pick up that chocolate, eat one apple instead!
>
> No fancy diets involved. No commercial stuff, no trendy stuff, nothing but my own willpower.
>
> Do it for seven days. Check your weight only at the start and the end, and nowhere in the middle. Once you truly understand the link between calories and weight (and you have your seven day log) your life will change forever! I was 60 years old before I tried this, and it actually sunk in immediately. I wish I had understood this fully, 30 years earlier.

My running helps me lose weight in any case. I know that, because my log has the raw data going back twenty years. It also shows that when I fall off the wagon and stop running, the weight all piles back on again.

Never before have I lost so much weight in such a short time. You'll know from the start of this book that one of the reasons I took up running was to get my weight under control. And it wasn't until 19 years after I started to be health conscious, that I actually struck upon the guaranteed way to lose weight.

After the first three weeks spanning part of June and July 2023 (when I lost 2.5kg) I promptly stopped the food diary and the calorie counting. In that three week window I had already become acutely aware of what I was eating and how many calories different types of food contain. The running log tells me that in the next three weeks I lost only 1kg. I had maintained the same amount of running, and in spite of being better educated and more conscientious about my food intake, the rate of weight loss was less than half of what it had been in the previous three weeks.

I started calorie counting again on 30 Jul 2023 and in the space of one further week I lost 1kg. This is it. This is the painful realisation that *weight management* is easier done by simply restricting energy consumption than by working hard at appropriate energy expenditure.

Dr Giles Yeo puts it most succinctly in his book when he says (somewhere right in the middle):

> *"The only way to gain weight is to eat more than you burn, and the only way to lose weight is to burn more than you eat. It is a fundamental law of physics, and there is no way of getting around it."*

He then goes on to explain how every fad diet works, because it simply addresses the fundamental law of physics, by disguising the real science in fancy dress.

Most importantly, what matters is *what* you eat. It matters more than your exercise routine. Why has it taken me years and years before I found people who laid it out in such simple, easy to understand terms? Yeo adds "you cannot outrun a bad diet".

I listened to Yeo deliver a lecture at The Royal Institution on 13 Aug 2021. A few days after that I bought his book, meaning to read it straight way, but it sat on the shelf. Two years after that, on 14 Jun 2023 I met Trembath. After meeting Trembath I finally start reading Yeo's book. Commencing on 14 Aug and finishing on 31 Oct 2023. It's an eye opener. It's entertaining, witty, and in places it's deeply scientific. It appears to contain some undergraduate degree level Biology. Even though I gave up Biology after 'O' Level, I read the book conscientiously and I filled in the gaps in my knowledge (of micro cellular biology) by studying some deeply technical stuff online.

I've mentioned BMI a few times in previous chapters, and we all know that BMI is flawed. But it's one of the simplest ways for us to get a handle on our weight gain or loss. You can do the more accurate DEXA (Dual-energy X-ray absorptiometry) if you want to. But you cannot do it with your tape measure and your bathroom scales at home. You'll need to engage professionals, go to their clinic, and pay them a lot of money to get a slightly better picture than the one that BMI gives you anyway. The point of DEXA is to measure your bone density. The side effect of DEXA is that it generates a "fat shadow" and that shadow can be analysed to help you understand the ratio of fat to other soft tissue. It's the preferred system for body builders because the shadow can distinguish between muscle and fat. If I were you, I'd just stick with BMI. I don't want to know my muscle to fat to bone ratios. I just want to know if I have a healthy weight.

Over the course of a six months during 2023 I lost 18% of my body weight. My BMI went down from 29.6 to 24.3, the lowest it had been since I was a twenty something. In case you've forgotten, I'm now 61.

There was some weight loss before my first marathon, and before my second marathon. But it didn't happen in any kind of significant, planned way. Not like the weight loss over those six months in 2023.

Chocolate

Try calorie counting, instead of trying the quick fixes that a lot of people reach for.

As I describe what happens next please imagine this, full size, on a plate in front of you. How many calories are there in an average tomato? And in 100g of cucumber? Your imaginary plate has an average tomato and a 10cm length from your average cucumber. What you have in front of you are 16 + 16 = 32 calories.

To be honest, it would be a lot easier just to reach for that bar of Cadbury's Dairy Milk chocolate and break off a strip (or two). Now imagine that chocolate. In one single segment, not a whole row with four segments, just in one single segment of Cadbury's Dairy Milk chocolate, there are 32 calories.

Same calories, tomato plus cucumber, or one segment of chocolate. Now ask me which one I'd opt for. Which one would you choose? I'm not your mum!

In the past I had a tendency to reach for the chocolate and break off one row of four segments. That totals 128 calories. Equally, I could have opened the salad draw, selected five tomatoes and one entire cucumber and eaten all of that instead, because that also totals 128 calories.

Which one would be better for me? That salad stuff alone gets me beyond my "five fruits and vegetables every day". It's also more nutritious and more satiating. The important word is "satiating". Things are not the same with ultra processed food like chocolate. Ultra processed food, according to van Tulleken, is the sort of thing that cannot be produced in the average domestic kitchen. It needs sophisticated commercial equipment. In his book *Ultra Processed Food* van Tulleken quotes Raube saying that "ultra processed food is not food, it's an industrially produced edible substance".

Yeo explains that the body digests ultra processed food very easily. And very quickly. You feel satiated for a moment and then it wears off. Whereas natural food, with a bit more bulk, and a lot more fibre, sticks around for longer. In my "four segments of chocolate" example you get the same 128 calories as with the plate full of tomatoes and cucumber. But the fresh food sticks around for longer, drip feeding you the calories over an hour or two, and providing you with fibre. Fibre cannot be digested and just passes through you. Those two factors contribute to feeling satiated - digestible ordinary food stays as food for longer, and indigestible fibre stays for as long as it takes to get rid of it.

Try feeding me three rows of chocolate (no, please don't try it in real life) and I could surely eat a fourth row. Try feeding me three whole cucumbers and I would probably say no to eating a fourth!

Take another example. The standard Mars Bar. How many calories are there in a 51g Mars Bar? Yes, there are 228 calories. For that, I could have one banana and ten strawberries added to an ample serving of 100g of fat free natural yoghurt.

People who cannot find time to prepare natural food will obviously reach for the quick and easy alternatives. Food retailers know this, which is why they put the chocolate (and not the tomatoes) next to the supermarket checkouts.

I'm not judging anyone. Remember what Confucius said:

> *"Discipline is just choosing between what you want now and want you want most."*

People who manage to lose weight are the people who woke up one day, and finally addressed the unpalatable reality that we are what we eat. Maybe it's worth a few more minutes each day to prepare fresh food? If you're aiming to spend a long time running long distances, then what's a few more minutes at meal time?

Eating lots of fresh food, and minimising processed and ultra processed food, helps me stay trim. With fruit and veg the easy advice is to "eat all the colours". With meat etc, there are reasons to minimise the intake of red meat, in favour of fish or poultry. The bibliography lists lots of resources, including van Tulleken and Yeo.

You cannot outrun a bad diet.

My Breakfast

I found that reducing breakfast cereal, and doing more egg on toast (nice granary bread with proper butter) led to a marked reduction in my calorie intake. If I reduce the bread and butter, and have more fruit instead, then the calorie count goes down even more.

Before the Geneva Marathon in 2018 my regular breakfast was a massive bowl of Alpen with semi skimmed milk, and one piece of fruit. By 2023 it had changed to one poached egg on toast, along with two types of fruit added to a small bowl of yoghurt.

Your toaster might have two slots in it. I have discovered that you can put just one piece of bread into just one of the slots! And still make toast! Who knew? Half of my bread and butter consumption has been eliminated.

Your Breakfast

I can't tell you the calorie count for your breakfast, you'll have to go and do this one yourself. I find that a calculator, a kitchen scale of the digital kind, and a pencil and paper are the best weight loss tools out there.

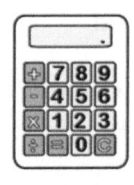

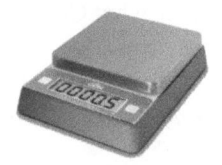

I have never followed a commercial diet or a trendy diet.

Take your regular cereal bowl and weigh it when it's empty. Now fill it with your regular breakfast cereal. How much does the cereal weigh? Calculate the calories from the chart on the packet.

Now, with the full bowl still on the scale, add in some milk. Now what does it weigh? Calculate the weight of the milk (1g = 1cc = 1ml) and then calculate the calories, again by referring to the little chart on the side of the milk carton. Total up all the calories.

Alternatively, get your box of eggs, your loaf of bread, and your butter (other types of spread are available). Look at the packets, how many calories are there in one egg plus one slice of bread plus one careful layer of spread? With just a little care, I can make 5g of butter cover one piece of toast. Do your calculations with a larger figure for the spread if that's the way you like to slap it on your toast.

You only have to measure each meal once, and then keep a note. I've given up with Alpen, I make my own home made muesli from separate foodstuffs, and I use a smaller cereal bowl than before. With a piece of fruit in both cases, my muesli breakfast has 545 calories. Compare that to my egg on toast breakfast which has 427 calories. The egg breakfast has 22% fewer calories.

I was astonished to see the difference between my breakfast of cereal and the breakfast with one poached egg. If you fry your egg you'll need to add in some more calories for the oil. I need just one tablespoon of olive oil to fry one egg, and I assume that half of the oil is left behind, meaning that I consume the other half. That's 10g of oil in the frying pan at the start, and by the end it's probably 5g of oil all over my egg. I end up ingesting 40 calories from the 5g of oil! I could have had one segment of chocolate and consumed fewer calories than in half a tablespoon of olive oil!

Now that you know *your* figures for *your* breakfast, you will probably want to know how many calories *you* burn when *you* run?

Put it another way, if I know that I burn X calories by running Y kilometres, then I will have do that N times per week in order to keep things in balance.

You can make this as scientific as you like, and you'll become a highly competitive runner. I don't want perfect charts, perfect schedules, and the perfect forecasting models that the professionals use. I just want a rule of thumb.

A Rule of Thumb

Use the online *Distance and Calorie Converter*.

Distance and Calorie Converter
www.dailycaloriescalculator.com

In my case, at my 2023 weight (and using both my distance and my running time) I burn 82 calories per kilometre. I burnt more when I was fatter, because I was carrying more weight around. As I get slimmer, the calories per kilometre are going down.

Translating that to match the distances I run, and I'm going to need almost 3,500 calories to get me through a marathon.

km	10	15	20	21.097	25	30	35	42.195
calories	823	1,235	1,647	1,659	2,058	2,470	2,881	3,455

The BBC has a useful guesstimator which tells you how many calories you need.

Calorie Guide
www.bbc.co.uk/food

How many calories? The NHS says "on average 2,500 per day for men, and 2,000 per day for women".

I'm smaller than average, and nowadays I'm much lighter than average. The BBC calculation says that without any exercise I need 1,805 calories per day. If I do my minimum level of running, that's 7 + 7 + 10 = 24k each week, then I've worked out that I need a daily average of 2,079 calories. Far, far less than the NHS recommended figures.

The NHS recommended figures are an average. Imagine a picture of Laurel & Hardy. Neither of them is average. One needs more than the average 2,500 calories per day, and the other needs less. I'm not average either! If I aim to adopt the average figure for anything, then one way or another I'm doing myself a disservice.

Bread

Bread is a big issue is the western world. It's one of the Ultra Processed Foods that van Tulleken recognises is a hard for us to eliminate. When I'm in the UK I each my fair share of bread, and a measure of cooked rice. When I'm in Japan it's the other way around, more rice than bread. Note that my own bathroom scales are part of my running kit and so they go on holiday with me! My Sunday weigh-ins show that my weight loss in Japan is always better than my weight loss in the UK.

Bread helps you put on too much weight too quickly. I rest my case.

Blood Pressure

For years I had high blood pressure, and I declined medication, vowing to control it myself with exercise and diet. More than twenty years ago I bought my own sphygmomanometer. I've recently bought my third one. With weekly use they each seem to last me about nine years. I have also (and only recently) brought my blood pressure down to acceptable levels. That correlates to the significant loss of weight in 2023.

Had I been on medication I would never have had the incentive to work hard on my health and fitness. The drugs would have masked the true picture, and I wouldn't have known what I was achieving by myself. The UK press keeps reminding us that obesity is a big problem. Research done by Howard in 2012 was reported in The Economist:

> *"Greater wealth means that bicycles are abandoned for motorbikes and cars, and work in the fields is swapped for sitting at a desk. In rich countries the share of the population that gets insufficient exercise is more than twice as high as in poor ones."*

The research goes on to say (in the Britain of 2012) that 25% of all women were obese, with men following close behind at 24%. On average, increased obesity leads to increased blood pressure.

The UK press doesn't help with depicting what "obese" actually looks like. They always seems to show images of people with "morbid obesity" and a BMI in excess of 40. It would be more helpful if they could show cases where the BMI is 31 or 32 and then we might gain a better understanding of what it actually looks like to be "obese". I'm guessing that a majority of the Members of Parliament that I see on TV news items are obese. That gives you some idea of was "obese" really looks like.

This is my understanding of the correlation between weight and blood pressure. It's not entirely scientific, and I am wholly unqualified to offer this explanation. It's my personal recollection of the "grapefruit story" that I came across when I worked at the British Medical Association in the 1990s.

> **The Humble Hard Working Grapefruit**
>
> Clench your fist. How big is it? The size of an average grapefruit? *Your* fist approximates to the size of *your* heart. Once you reach adulthood, your heart doesn't grow any bigger. It might become more efficient and more effective if you take up aerobic exercise, but as with your height, your heart is not really going to grow any more over your adult life.
>
> That heart has to service 100% of your body. The bigger your body, the more effort the same sized heart has to put in. If your heart cannot expand as much as your waist line, then all it can do is pump more blood more quickly, or pump it harder. And the harder it works at pumping blood around your increasingly large body, the higher your blood pressure has to be.

I cannot quote the sources from the 1990s, because I cannot remember them, and I have no written records from back then. I would be happy to find any research proving or disproving this theory. I can assure you that I've been down that rabbit hole, I've looked, I cannot find the supporting research, but then again, I do not have a paid subscription to The British Medical Journal, nor The Lancet, nor any other medical material.

Putting on weight caused my blood pressure to go up. Losing weight made it go down. I have twenty years of records on my running log to back this up.

Health is Threat Management

Excess weight is a threat. High blood pressure is a threat. Thanks to Dr Georges Canguilhem, Professor Richard Trembath and Dr Giles Yeo, I now manage these threats with some effectiveness.

"Health is threat management, and the ability to adapt to one's environment."

You have to count the calories, or your fancy commercial diets will continue to reward the aggressive commercial operators who want to continually sell you their commercial products. A diet only works if you stick to it. You can either keep buying the commercial solution (that's what they want you to do) or you can adapt your natural diet to banish the unhelpful foods. Sorry Alpen, banished!

Or try the new wave of slimming drugs? It's the same commercial trick. The drugs only work while you're taking (and paying for) the drugs.

You are what you eat, so eat healthy!

Clothing

It's great losing weight. Although the one big drawback is that you need to buy new clothes. My entire wardrobe was replaced in 2023 and 2024. Professional, casual and sporting wear. Remember what I said in Chapter 3 about wearing kit which was too big, XL or XXL? It's all gone. Now that I have the right physique, the older stuff has all been replaced by size M.

Chapter 12 - Books, Books and More Books

Life Long Learning

There are hundreds and thousands of books about running. Some of them specifically about marathons. I bought a couple through Amazon. They were disappointing. Both very superficial, and neither of them had an index at the back.

One day, I spent an afternoon in a book shop and then a library, leafing through a number of running books. It surprised me that only 10% of them had an index! Of that, only half of those indexes contained entries with either "fartlek" or "interval training". There's an index at the back of this book. And there's a bibliography too, listing all the materials which have helped me.

In contrast to the bland ones, the books by Cory Wharton-Malcolm (personal trainer) and by Paul Olima (professional football player) were really helpful. They were about fitness in general, not only about running, and they each devoted a few paragraphs to interval training.

Even more helpful was John Shepherd (athlete & coach, long jump & triple jump). His book has a good discussion spread across several pages, covering interval training and lactate. It has some of the science, and some of the detailed explanations that I wanted. Shepherd explains the "why" when many others don't.

There's only so much time and money that I can devote to reading. A bit like having time available to run, or money to spend on shoes, shoes and more shoes! Everything is a compromise. My collection of books, books and more books is a compromise. This book you're reading right now is a compromise. There are limits to how much I can study, and how much I can write!

Students & Teachers

When I was a teacher from 1999 to 2002, the expression "life long learning" was touted around without being particularly well defined.

In its most recent 2019 incarnation, the UK government talks about:

> *"every student, with the aptitude and the desire, getting the support they need to pursue higher level learning".*

That's from the Augar Report which coincidentally was prepared by a panel of experts from my old Uni, King's College London.

The Augar Report
kclpure.kcl.ac.uk/portal

However, that definition is *not* what KCL taught me twenty years earlier. I had learnt that life long learning was for *everybody*, not just students. The mentors told us that by using our (mythical, magical) teaching powers, we would instil the concept of "life long learning" in *everybody*, in order to encourage *everybody* to aspire to greater knowledge. It's related to what Plato calls "the divided line of knowledge".

In my opinion "the divided line" is really a "ladder" of knowledge. Divided in the sense that you can progress from one step to another if that's what you want to do. Climb up or down as far as you like, for as long as it's helpful, and improving the quality of your life. Everybody has their own limit. I've not yet reached mine.

A better definition of "life long learning" from Salford University is:

> *"the ongoing, voluntary, and self motivated pursuit of learning for either personal or professional reasons"*

That is very much in line with what I discuss in this chapter. Personally, I want to live longer and not kill myself, and I want to learn more about how to do that. Michael Greger even wrote a book called "How not to die" though it's about nutrition, not running.

Rewards

I don't necessarily agree with this next quote, but my friend John will tell you:

> *"You should live your life like a ride on a rollercoaster, finally sliding sideways into your grave, your body thoroughly used up and worn out, strawberries and cream in one hand, a glass of champagne in the other, screaming woo hoo, let's go around again!"*

My personal vision is a little more restrained, and you'll read about that later. Although I do like to have a good measure of dopamine sometimes. I don't think I'd like it all day, every day, and shorten my life in the process. The point of telling you this is that everything is a trade off.

Here's what another friend Simon has to say about trade offs:

> *"the reward for doing it has to be better than the reward for not doing it, otherwise people will simply not do it"*

And there you have the crux of the exercise/fitness/running problem. The reward for doing it is something intangible which you hope to experience in your future. The reward for not doing it is that you can indulge in all the fun stuff you like, right now, even if it's not healthy.

Didn't Canguilhem say something about that? Threat management?

This is the "deferred gratification" dilemma, made all the more difficult by not knowing exactly what your deferred gratification is going to look like. It's a complex subject, and if you want to explore it in detail you might like to start with "psychological health". Although that's a difficult area to study without getting bogged down in lots of texts discussing distressing mental health issues in general.

So here's one example of something that has helped me.

A Food Diary

There have been two or three times when my younger self read articles in newspapers or magazines, which extolled the virtues of maintaining a food diary. My younger self did it, and it was mind numbingly dull each time. After a week of recording everything, I had a list of food and drink. The only bit that sort of made sense was the list of alcoholic drinks, which I could convert to units, which (in the 1990s and early 2000s) I could compare to NHS guidance about the recommended intake.

I had no figures for the quantity of food, nor the calorie count, because none of those worthy newspaper articles explained enough about how or why the food diary should be maintained. On each of those occasions one week of tedious effort had led to nothing. My "psychological health" didn't really improve. If anything, the thought crossed my mind "well that was a waste of time".

For a number of reasons I eventually gave up alcohol, but not until 1 Feb 2004. That was more than a year before my general health and fitness drive really took off. After that my psychological health definitely improved, and presumably there was at least some correlation between my earlier, abandoned food diaries and the later change in my alcohol consumption.

I had demonstrated to myself that I had understood what Confucius had said and I was heading in the right direction.

> *"Discipline is just choosing between what you want now and want you want most."*

Simply *knowing* that I could change my habits was boosting my psychological health. Having done it once before with alcohol, the same psychological boost happened again (many years later) in 2023 when I started counting calories and really lost some weight.

And here's the crux. In the weeks when I conscientiously recorded calorie consumption, I was deliberately selective about the things I was eating, and I lost weight effectively. In the weeks when I was merely *mindful* of the calories, and worked with vague ideas about limiting consumption (but recorded nothing in writing) weight loss happened but to a much lesser extent.

I learnt that I can lose weight more effectively when I count calories than when I don't. That was a stunning psychological health boost! Not only do I know how to do it, I know that I can do it, and that it leads to tangible results within days. I routinely log my weight every Sunday morning and I've been doing that for years. I could see the weight loss, evidenced on the bathroom scales. I cannot over emphasise the importance of keeping a written log.

If you don't measure it you don't manage it!

The Power of the Written Word

Without a written log of my running, my injuries, and my calorie consumption, I would not have learnt so much so quickly. Without a written plan, I wouldn't have achieved as much as I have. What does your plan say? Your rudimentary version of Appendix One? Not mine!

Underpinning it all, my plan says that I want to live longer and not kill myself. That's the simple answer. There is no need to run marathons nor even 10k. Lots of people live a long and healthy life without ever running very far.

There will come a day when I don't run any more. Perhaps in my 70s or 80s or 90s. I don't know when, but I do know that it will leave a gaping void in my life. When I can no longer run, I will address that with a daily walk to the shops. My local supermarket is 1.5k from my home. I can take a nice circular 4k route, doing 2.5k outbound followed by 1.5k inbound carrying the bags of shopping. And I won't need to carry much if I adopt a daily shopping routine.

I will however, continue to do my twice yearly visit to the 400m track. And log my performance over six laps, whether I run, or walk, or shuffle.

If all else fails, instead of six laps of the track I will walk 1200m from my home, turn around and walk 1200m back, time the journey, and log it. And when I can no longer do that I will be an extremely old man.

I have learnt the value of keeping a log.

Energy Management

In order to extract the maximum value from my log I did a recap of my previous races. Marathon 1 Milton Keynes, and Marathon 2 Geneva. Although I didn't do that detailed recap until 18 days before Marathon 3 Chelmsford!

In each of my first two marathons I hit the *precursor* to hitting the wall. I simply hadn't realised it at the time! I hadn't "hit the wall" in the classic sense, because my body kicked in with its inbuilt protection system, a self defence mechanism which subconsciously had told me what to do.

I may not have wanted it, nor intended it, but intuitively I did the right thing. I slowed down. In Milton Keynes I resorted to some walking after 21k, and finally lay down on the grass for around five minutes at about the 30k mark. In Geneva, I had unexpectedly switched from running to walking (briefly) at the 25k mark. In both cases, I had run for at least half the route, and in both cases I completed the full marathon with my habitual system of yomping.

What I did was just enough to stave off the classic "hitting the wall". I did *not* suffer a complete and instant loss of energy, and I did not collapse in a heap on the road having used up all of my available energy stores.

When I look back at all the long training runs over the years, (about two dozen of them, at 25k and more) my log shows that in the majority of cases I have notes that mention fatigue from the 20k mark or later. That all coincides with two hours or more of running. One unforgettable experience was running up a gentle, but long ascent in *Ferney Voltaire* in early 2018, with snow on the ground, and nearing the 30k mark of my training run. I simply stopped. Not instantly, not abruptly, but purposefully and conscientiously I decided to stop.

I sat down on a dwarf wall at the front of somebody's garden. Then I lay down on the snow covered grass verge, feet up the slope, head down, just as I had done in Milton Keynes. Snow be damned! I was fatigued beyond belief, and if I wanted to lie down on snow that's fine! It's better than sitting on a freezing cold, snow covered, concrete wall! My body's inbuilt self defence mechanism obviously told me when it was time to get up, because the slow walk home was a better option than continuing to lie down in the snow.

Whether it's the precursor, or the full monty, the solution to hitting the wall is simple. Lower the intensity, in one of two ways:

- stop and rest, or
- slow down drastically.

That explains why so many people end up walking the final stages of a marathon. Their bodies have an inbuilt mechanism that stops them from risking collapse. You can override that mechanism if you have the willpower, although these days we rarely hear stories of people falling over from exhaustion.

Better still, do some advance preparation. Prevention is better than cure! Do some carb loading beforehand, and consume energy supplements throughout the race.

What's the average time to finish a marathon? According to data collected since 2001, the UK average is 4 hours 37 minutes. A lot of people are faster than that, and that means that a lot of people are slower! In the UK and the USA marathons have become a mass participation sport with more people than ever doing them, regardless of their ability.

Prior to 2001 the average was 4 hours 28 minutes.

Prior to 1986 the average was 3 hours 52 minutes.

In the past people might only enter a marathon if they were capable of running half decent times. Now it's certainly a much wider playing field. The average times in Germany and Spain are better, because they have fewer participants from the general public.

Broadly speaking, the human body has enough glycogen to keep you going for about two hours continuously. Glycogen is the readily available sugar, small local stores in your muscles, special fatty deposits around the liver, and some travelling around constantly in the blood stream. There's a bit of glycogen everywhere. A higher than normal energy requirement will mean that the local stores in the muscles are used first and are depleted quickly. Then the supplies in the blood, and then around the liver.

Once the glycogen has gone, you need to get more energy from somewhere. In basic terms your body starts to eat itself, using a process called gluconeogenesis. Finally the body says "no" to the desire to cannibalise muscle in order to make that very same muscle work, and that's when you hit the wall in the worst possible way. Runners who pull every last energy resource from their body simply collapse as their legs will carry them no further.

Carb Loading

Eventually, I realised that I was fighting two different battles.

I had heard about carb loading in the past. When I was carrying excess weight I really wasn't interested in carrying more carbs! I didn't know that the objective of carb loading was to promote bountiful glycogen stores. I had mistakenly thought that carb loading was going to add more adipose tissue. And yes, indiscriminate consumption of carbs will eventually lead to more fat. Done properly, carb loading is about getting the right balance, more glycogen and stopping short of more adipose tissue. As a uneducated beginner, I didn't want to be fatter so I didn't carb load.

My original objective in 2005 was to lose weight. My objective in 2024 was to run continuously for 42k without resorting to walking. They are two different and unrelated goals, albeit with a bit of overlap.

Losing weight requires one type of plan. Running a marathon (without walking bits of it) requires a distinctly different sort of plan. It took me many years before I worked that out!

By October 2024 my BMI was 22.4 and so, before the race, I needed to augment my in-built stores of carbohydrate. That would provide me with more readily available glycogen.

Start adding more carbs to your diet about two weeks before marathon day. Slowly at first, and then build it up a bit more in the last few days before the race. If you're following a strict diet, pause it for two weeks. You can resume afterwards. Taking two weeks out of your year to eat normally is not going to fundamentally impede your diet, but it is going to fundamentally improve your welfare on a marathon.

Normal eating means be "normal". Don't overdose on ice cream! Do have rice or pasta or potatoes with your meals.

I started having cereal for breakfast, rather than egg on toast. I also willingly added some marmalade to my toast! And a chocolate bar or two. Not on the toast I hasten to add! Sometimes I ate toast and marmalade. At other times I ate some chocolate!

My wife, delighted by the opportunity to do some home baking (after a long hiatus) fed me apple pies topped with whipped cream, and chocolate sponge cakes and all sorts of fancy things. Just for that two week period.

I didn't overdose on sugar and I still lost weight during those two weeks, mainly because I was having small portions of dessert, and I was still doing my long runs on Sundays!

It was the fact that I studied the science that made the big difference. I honestly did not know that the body cannot metabolise fat fast enough to keep up with high intensity exercise. It needs glycogen. As soon as it notices the extra demand for energy the body *does* begin to work on metabolising fat as well. Typically that starts after about twenty minutes, but the body is not capable of doing enough, quickly enough, without some help. Lowering the intensity of your running to the "fat max" level (the aerobic threshold or AeT) will help establish a balance between the energy that comes from glycogen and from fat.

Adequate Preparation

In Chapter 11 the online *Distance and Calorie Converter* was mentioned, and I added that in my case I burn 82 calories per kilometre. I also know from Yeo's book that one gram of fat equates to roughly nine calories. Assuming that my metabolism can work fast enough, then 400g of body fat is more than enough to see me through a marathon. But human metabolism *doesn't* work that fast!

The solution is energy gel (other supplements are available).

Without the internet, and places like The Royal Institution, and a vast array of authors still publishing books, I would never have been able to work all this out. Life long learning in my case has never stopped.

Interval Training

Initially I could not understand why the "how to" guides and the marathon plans were all placing so much emphasis on *interval training*.

The guides consistently tell you "what" to do and fail to tell you "why" you should do it. I had absolutely no intention of running a marathon in bursts of sprints intermingled with slow running. I do not expect to be running up flights of stairs in a stadium as part of my marathon. What is the point of *interval training* I thought? I was planning to run a marathon at a steady pace, and that's what the "how to" guides generally advocate.

For years (twenty years almost) I was dismissive of the idea of interval training. It was only after I looked up the Swedish word *fartlek* that I began to understand. And it was a bit too late in the day for me to do much about it. Then I found John Shepherd's material and he explained "why".

This is why you should do interval training . . .

It improves the body's ability to convert sugars and fat into energy, and you'll develop bigger, better muscles, with bigger, better glycogen stores!

We're not talking about body builder proportions. What we're talking about is augmenting what you have, as best you can, to make things a bit easier on yourself. Do nothing special, and your glycogen stores will be nothing special. Do something about muscle size and strength, and you will be helping yourself.

Proper interval training is not an activity to be tackled if you're a complete beginner. You need to steadily build up your ability. Once you're comfortable with running modest distances, set aside a different day to try some interval training instead. You'll end up promoting more lactic acid, and you'll begin to build a tolerance to it. And you'll develop bigger, better muscles which can oxidise fuel more quickly and more effectively. That enables you to perform better.

Health and Fitness and Diet

So overall, the key things are health and fitness and diet. There is no need for me to actually do another marathon.

What this adventure has taught me is that we have to be masters of change. I learnt that the web is fluid, that WalkJogRun changed hands, that materials disappeared, and that the Runners World forecasting tool was taken down because it was inaccurate. All of that taught me to copy and paste useful material. My wiki has links to articles on The Guardian, The Times, The Economist and The Lancet, and to nearly all of the races I've done. I've copied and pasted some of the best material (for my own personal education) in case any of the originals vanish!

> *Change is inevitable. Except from a vending machine.*

The first half marathon I ever did was in Folkestone. The website is no longer there. The results have gone. The marathon routes for Milton Keynes and

Geneva have changed since I did them. Though fortunately I did take screen shots of the old websites back in the day, and on my wiki I can see the precise routes that I followed. Had I known all of this twenty years ago I would have been far more meticulous keeping records of everything that I'd seen and done.

The wiki also has pages for the luminaries . . .

- Dr Georges Canguilhem
- Prof Richard Trembath
- Dr Giles Yeo

. . . and it shows me the personal notes I took, and refers me to related online resources. Like a one hour YouTube video of Yeo addressing The Royal Institution. I cannot emphasise enough how important these three people have been to me, and I wish that I had come across their work earlier. My plan was to run a marathon, but the overriding dream was to lose some weight and to become fitter and healthier.

- Canguilhem told me what to do (in 2021)
- Trembath told me why I should do it (in 2023)
- Yeo told me how it's done (in 2021)

Crucially, Trembath kindled the "aha moment" when he described a restaurant menu to me. The cheese board had a note saying 1,200 calories. It was the highest value for any of the desserts on the menu. That alone amounts to about half the daily recommended intake for an adult male!

I wanted to share with you the role played by these three healthcare specialists. That's because the KCL ethos has stayed with me. I continually like to do something "in service of society".

No matter how you interpret the concept of "life long learning", it is valuable.

Chapter 13 - The Secret Sauce

Making sense of it all

Please resist the temptation to read this chapter first. If you haven't done the preceding chapters in the order in which they are laid out, then this chapter on its own is not going to make a whole lot of sense!

I've been on this campaign for twenty years now, and nowhere on the web, nor in various books, nor in any dialogue, have I ever found "The Formula" which sets out clearly and concisely how to prepare for and run a marathon.

In this chapter I have done my best to create my own version of "The Formula". It's less about the detail of what running to do and when, as that's already the focus of many other resources. This one is more about strategy and planning, from an amateur point of view.

This is *Proactive Paul's Formula*, a rudimentary formula with some of the logic explained, and with a few personal anecdotes thrown in. You will have to build your own formula. Borrow some or all or none of mine if you wish!

It's not a secret!

The first thing to point out is that the secret sauce is not a secret. It's no doubt out there for everybody to find. It's just not particularly visible nor is it very well explained. It's omitted from every marathon resource I've ever read and it took me a long time to work it out for myself. Well, perhaps not work out all of it, but to work out enough of the formula to be able to boost my confidence significantly.

I had been on this path for twenty years, yet the murky jigsaw puzzle only began to fit together when the Chelmsford Marathon was just 18 days away.

The shock realisation would not have arrived if I had not been writing this book! A book about my third marathon, and a book which at that stage had absolutely no mention of "hitting the wall"! As you've already seen, Chapter 10 has a panel which discusses the ubiquitous wall. It was a late revision, added to the book in the final stages of drafting.

Hitting the wall? Was I at any time, at the risk of a complete and instant loss of energy?

Yes and no!

A Rudimentary Formula

The first few steps of this rudimentary formula relate to "running" in general. The later steps become more marathon specific.

Step 1
Start Early

Super heroes can adopt "the 16 week plan" which is a favourite recipe in the established "how to" guides. The ones that assume you're already a half decent runner in your twenties or thirties. Mere mortals like me should start long before that. Twelve months in advance (or more), not four months!

Over a lengthy training period you should concentrate on duration, not on distance. Learn how to run for hours on end.

Step 2
Set Goals

Have big goals and little goals, peppered throughout your training plan. Give yourself a variety of things to focus on.

When you're a beginner it's hard to know what the right sort of goal is. It doesn't matter! Set a goal anyway. You can always modify it later. Your earliest goals should already be written down somewhere. You did do the written exercise from Chapter One didn't you? Have another look at what your younger self wrote down. What exactly are you trying to do?

Step 3
Learn From Experience

Log everything. Plan, do, review. Inspect your log before each run. How did you get on last time? And the time before that? When I look back, going over one or two recent records helps me develop "the strategy for today".

On a regular basis (in my case that's once a week before my long Sunday run) spend a little more time looking back a bit further. And looking forward a little to the near future. For me that means comparing (for example) this 25k run with the last few 25k runs, comparing this one with the same one a year ago, or the same one five years ago.

Then I look at the second tab on my spreadsheet, the bit that outlines the collection of the next set of training runs. Right now, where am I in this ideal line of progression? What am I going to do differently today? What issue am I going to focus on?

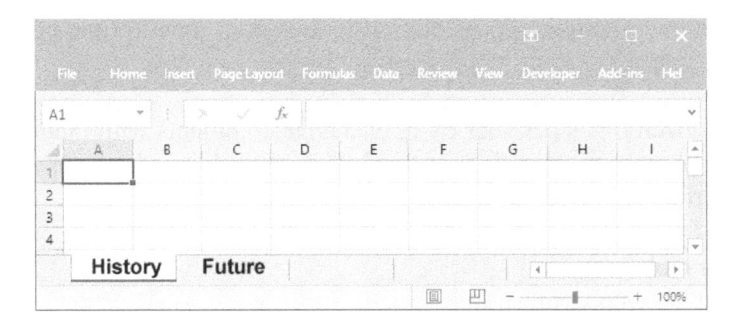

If my notes say "set off too fast", or "walked a bit after 16k" then I pick one or two things to work on "today". Trying to get the right pace, or trying to reach the 17k waypoint before resorting to any walking. The mantra in my head goes "no more walking" or "pick up the pace Paul" or "power through it". In my repertoire I have a dozen expressions which I call upon when needed.

Sometimes I have a little angel who rides quietly on my left shoulder. Her name is Prudence, and she only ever says one word, whispering a soft, gentle, comforting "prudence". Reassuring me that there are good reasons why I never run up and down steps. Warning me at the places where I've injured myself in the past, of the known defects in paved surfaces. Warning me at the ridiculous 90° corners at the Oxo Tower and the passage below Westminster Bridge.

Over the years I have conjured up lots of things, peculiar mantras, crazy imagery and weird motivational concepts. It all helps to add variety to the journey. I don't listen to music when I run. I listen to the things happening around me, the noise of the traffic, the footsteps of the faster runner catching up with me from behind, the occasional screaming toddler. Even if I can't see these things I know what's going on around me, and it helps with anticipating any problems. When I feel like I need to have a bit of music, I silently hum in my head the theme tune from Chariots of Fire:

"Da da da da dum dah!"

I make up fictitious characters for the people I see, like *The Harlem Shuffler* and *Mr Last Orders*. They're were all listed for your amusement back on page 84. I also recognise a lot of the road sweepers and the security officers who work along my regular training routes. When the chance presents itself easily, I say "good morning" to them.

Step 4
Smile

Make people happy. Smile at them, greet them, making others happy makes you happy. Not everybody you pass obviously, but from time to time engage with the people you see.

At least a dozen times per year I will exchange comments with random people at special photo opportunities, somebody in a wedding dress, or somebody wearing a robe and a mortar board:

- You look gorgeous!
- That's a wonderful smile!
- Congratulations!

If it's another runner who's having a bit of a flaky moment:

- You've done well, keep smiling!
- You're doing well, keep it up!
- Keep smiling, it makes it easier!

Or when I see a runner on a mission:

- Impressive stuff!
- Good pace!

Not everybody, not every time. But sometimes! If the runner is wearing earphones I know it'll only add to their concern if I try to engage them with pleasantries, so these comments are only delivered when I think the moment feels right.

Over time, I've come to recognise one or two other runners on my regular routes, and occasionally I'll offer a cheery "good morning". If anybody greets me first, runner or not, I always try to reply.

Uniquely, I sometimes greet people with "welcome to The Lake District". Notably, to some of the participants on the overnight "Shine" walking marathon which Cancer Research UK runs every September. They're still walking when the sun comes up. Anybody who knows what the South Bank looks like after a night of heavy rain will know exactly what I'm talking about! It has more lakes than The Lake District. Giving a smile, and certainly getting a smile in return, does wonders for morale. You're trying to make this whole running experience more pleasant, not see it as some kind of torture!

Step 5
Build a Routine

Humans are creatures of habit, so let's form some good habits! Many habits are second nature. Debra Kawahara PhD says it's quite possible that we don't even recognise some of the habitual actions which make up our day. They become a large part of who we are over time. Bad habits certainly work like that!

As runners, we need our *good habits* to become second nature. Once they're formed, the part of the brain that was needed to focus on developing them is then freed up so that we can focus on other things.

In the early days I used to go out running whenever I could spare the time. Morning, afternoon, or evening. It took a while to build my routine of 6.00am starts, three times per week. Evening runs were abandoned after my first summer in Switzerland, because it was simply too hot. Mornings became a habit

And when I vowed "no more running in the dark and no more injuries" it became a little hard to adjust to "waiting for sunrise" before going out. But it developed into a good habit. As winter set in, my running meant more and more intrusion into "commuter time" and that meant that I was sometimes running amongst jumbled groups of pedestrians. Quite dense groups on the approaches to some railway stations. So, I worked on changing my mindset. Slowing down for pedestrians was a price I should learn to accept when running later than usual. In exchange, I knew that I had reduced the risk of hitting unseen objects in the dark, and causing lower limb injuries.

How long does it take to form a new habit?

Sixty six days. On average!

That's according to Phillippa Lally PhD, a health psychology researcher at University College London. In 2010 her work showed that it took anywhere from 18 days to 254 days for people to form a new habit. The average was 66 days. Her research built on the earlier work of Dr Maxwell Maltz whose 1960 book on Psycho-Cybernetics gave rise to the "21 Days" myth.

The "21 Days" myth spread quickly. It was easy to understand. The time frame is short enough to be inspiring and long enough to be believable. What he actually said was that it takes "a minimum of 21 days" to form a new habit.

You cannot automatically orchestrate life changing habits in the space of three weeks!

The upshot of all this is: try something new, really concentrate on it for the first 21 days otherwise it's likely to wither into insignificance. Get to 66 days and you can be pretty sure that you're nailing it. If by 254 days the new idea has not firmly taken root, then perhaps you might want to try a different strategy.

That's all the pontificating on habits that I can offer! It's backed by professional research which is all detailed in the bibliography.

The Half Marathon v The Marathon

A marathon is a completely different kettle of fish to a half marathon. To illustrate the magnitude of the difference between a marathon and a half marathon the best analogy I can give you is "meal time".

Imagine that running a 10k race is like preparing beans on toast for one. Relatively speaking, it's easy.

Imagine that running a half marathon is like preparing beans on toast for two. Roughly speaking it's about twice as demanding. Most people who can do the former, can also do the latter.

As I finished each of my early 10k races the thought crossed my mind that "I just need to do this twice, and that's about the effort needed for a half marathon". That's not too far from the truth. Twice the effort, or thereabouts. No doubt, many other runners have had that thought too.

No doubt, many other runners have also experienced the next seemingly obvious step. As I finished each of my half marathons I had foolishly thought that "I just need to do this twice, and that's about the effort needed for a full marathon".

Oh no it isn't!

Incidentally, I've met a few people who have categorically stated, after doing a half marathon, that they have absolutely no intention of "doing this twice".

In any case, it's not as simple as "doing this twice".

Imagine that running a full marathon is like preparing a three course roast dinner for four people. Roughly speaking it's about ten times as demanding as making beans on toast for one (or running a 10k). It is far, far harder than "doing a half marathon twice".

> The reasons are "human metabolism" and "energy consumption".
>
> It was only after reworking a draft version of this book that I revisited my aversion to using energy gel. After my experience in Milton Keynes I was totally dismissive of the idea of using energy gel. Before Chelmsford, I did my research, and gradually I became more accepting. And finally, I did a complete U turn! For anything that's longer than a half marathon you *have to* take energy supplements in order to cover the distance without interruption
>
> I didn't know this before, and that's why I spent my first two marathons learning "how not to run a marathon".
>
> Remember the analogy, the challenges are more like "beans on toast" and "beans on toast twice" and "a three course roast dinner for four".

Step 6
Study a Little Science

Psychology. Nutrition. Anatomy. Cell biology. There's no need to do any sub atomic particle physics unless you really want to!

In my school days I was good at physics and lousy at biology. Here was my chance to make up for the past. I was fascinated by mitochondria, the tiny organelles found within cells. Yeo introduced me to mitochondria and ATP in his book, and I went online in order to study all of this and more. All the marathon resources I had ever read had skipped over this vital issue. I learnt it from online resources for undergrads and postgrad students. Here's a simpler version of the relevant science . . .

Assuming that my metabolism can work fast enough, then 400g of body fat is more than enough (for somebody of my size) to complete a 42k run. But that doesn't mean that 400g of fat will see me through a marathon in one go. It will allow me to cover 42k only if I split it up into manageable chunks, over many, many hours.

A quick recap . . . that's because the body cannot metabolise fat as fast as the muscles can consume energy. As your glycogen stores begin to disappear, the body augments that automatically by starting to metabolise fat. Slowly at first, and then a little faster. But nowhere near fast enough to satisfy the energy hungry muscles during an actual marathon.

More info . . . most importantly, fat cannot be easily metabolised without the presence of muscle glycogen. Hence, if muscle glycogen levels are badly depleted, it doesn't matter that fat is available, it cannot be utilised effectively and that leads to a drastic drop in performance.

That's why it's important not to start too fast on long training runs, using up all your glycogen stores too quickly. In exercise lasting more than four hours, even protein can be broken down. Your muscles are basically masses of protein. Your body will cannibalise the muscle tissue itself in order to make the necessary glycogen for fuel. As a method of energy conversion it's extremely inefficient and it's the body's last resort for survival.

Step 7
The Secret Ingredient in the Secret Sauce

The secret ingredient in the secret sauce is energy gel!

It could be anything sugary to be honest, gel, chews, bars, drinks, or boiled sweets. If I had stuck with my boiled sweets strategy I would have needed to carry and consume 48 boiled sweets over one marathon. Or four packets at 100g a time. Crunching one sweet every 875 metres!

Now that I know this, my Geneva Marathon strategy of one sweet every 10k looks completely inept. Right idea, wrong implementation. My Milton Keynes Marathon strategy was even worse! No plan for any energy supplements at all, and one foolish experiment with one free gel sachet.

I didn't have the luxury of time to test out lots of new energy strategies. With 18 days to go, I bought a large multi pack of SIS Orange Energy Gels. They weigh 60g each and contain 22g of carbohydrate. It's recommended that you take three per hour. I will need 16 of them as I plan to complete a marathon in about 5 hours and 30 minutes.

Step 8
The Secret Strategy That Nobody Tells You

The secret strategy in the secret sauce is to carry your own larder!

The "how to" guides tell you to plan your marathon, noting where the water stations are, and planning how and when you're going take on energy gel. Astonishingly, at the same time (and without fail) these guides conveniently overlook the fact that when you do a long training run there are no water stations along your route.

That means that nobody is there to provide you with instalments of water, banana, orange, or energy gel. You're going to have to provide your own, and short of installing secret squirrel food stations along your route, that means that you're going to have to carry your own supplies. As I coined it, carry your own larder.

If you're going to do some running for anything over two hours then you're going to need to take energy supplements. Many a time I have done training runs of 25k, 30k and 35k. These days they all take me in excess of 3 hours. My cheap backpack is lovely, but it's not built for these long runs.

What I needed was a backpack with more pouches. Or a belt which is specially designed for carrying gel sachets. Belts like that are available. I've seen one or two in the past, big hefty runners wearing what look like ammunition belts laced with six or eight sachets. For a start, I don't want a military look, and for another thing, I need 16 gel sachets. So either I need one stupidly large belt or I need two normal ones.

I once saw a chap with two of these belts across his shoulders and chest, and he looked like the archetypal Mexican bandit. Or I needed a more sensible approach. And I needed it now (urgently, 18 days before Chelmsford) in order to quickly get used to training with a fully loaded larder!

That meant that I didn't have the luxury of enough time to buy a new backpack, or two, or three, until a process of trial and error helped me identify the right one for me. In any case, I had grown to like my stupid little backpack and the arrangement of goodies spread around its various pockets. I knew what was where and I knew how to find it when I needed it. All I needed were two extra pouches, carrying eight energy gel sachets each, attached to the front straps.

Looking around at home for suitable pouches I found velvet jewellery bags and I found two identical canvas pencil cases. The pencil cases were a little larger than they needed to be, but being fabric I could modify them, fold over one of the longer sides a little, sew that down, and then sew the pencil cases onto the front straps of the backpack. They had to go on at a bit of an angle, and a little high up, so that I could still use the other pockets, but that was OK.

Casting aesthetic niceties to one side, and sewing down each pouch in five places, the modified pencil cases did the job. To stop the jangle of metal on metal as I ran, the metal tabs on the zips were removed and replaced with string. The original loops guiding the water pipe were now hidden so I added some velcro loops (cable ties for computer stuff) to the top of the pouches

Instead of wearing two ammunition belts I now appeared to be wearing some sort of military webbing! Oh well, military look! Never mind, the time had come to try it out.

Step 9
Dress Rehearsals

In the final few weeks before the third marathon I had managed to slow my pace to a marathon pace. I had learnt to start slowly and I called it my "grandad pace". The pace sheet on my right wrist served as a reminder at every waypoint. The stopwatch on my left wrist was telling me that I was getting it right. I was consistently reaching my waypoints within ten seconds of my target time. Now, all I needed to do was achieve that whilst carrying a larder!

Although my modified backpack had space for 16 energy gel sachets, my first trial run required just nine. Twenty five kilometres, taking me just over three hours, where I would consume one sachet every 20 minutes, or more accurately, one sachet every 3k. I carried 16 in any case, just to check the viability of this new bit of kit.

That meant that I was carrying a heavy load. Sixteen gel sachets at 60g each, and about 1.5 litres of water, approaching nearly 2.5kg in all. I actually consumed less water than before, because the gel sachets were providing some of the liquids I needed.

The newly equipped backpack did the job! But I had nowhere to dispose of the waste! I carried empty sachets in my hand until I found a bin. I'm lucky that central London has litter bins in various places. After the first dress rehearsal, I added one more pouch, a smaller pencil case attached with velcro to one of the larger pencil cases. There are photos of the whole ugly assembly on my blog!

Backpack
www.dontreadmyblog.com

The smaller pencil case is exclusively for waste. On the second dress rehearsal the velcro separated due to movement. It was then gaffer taped to the larger one.

The "how to" guides tell you to you do your training the way you intend to do your marathon. Their complete failure to even mention carrying supplies, let alone discuss "how to" carry them, is simply beyond me!

You need to train. And you need to carry your own larder when you train. Or you'll need ten very understanding friends at strategic locations, to act as volunteer helpers!

Step 10
Add Variety

The biggest mistake I made in my training was to persistently aim for a decent speed and a decent distance. I had only one running system with one mindset. Marathon running requires various, complementary training routines.

My basic system worked fine when I was preparing for something as straight forward as a 10k race or a half marathon. Luckily, my half marathon times were little more than two hours, and my glycogen stores lasted the distance. Luckily I was able to cope with half marathons, by following my 10k strategy.

My training for full marathons would have gone a lot better if I had started adding in some variety and started doing that quite early in my program. Nobody explained this clearly enough. That's what I meant earlier when I said a lot of the advice I read was "superficial". What I needed were three different types of training run. There was no need to cover all the bases every time. And I needed to adopt a different mindset for each of type of run. That means having different days to work on a different focus.

- speed focus - shorter runs - the way you want to do a 10k race.
- muscle focus - interval training - completely unrelated to any speed objective or distance objective - the objective is to strengthen your muscles.
- marathon focus - longer runs - endurance and stamina, aiming to find your steady marathon pace over a long distance.

It was a bit too late in the day for me to adopt a mixed routine. I could either do the Chelmsford Marathon 2024 on the basis of the training I had already done, or I could take a further six months to prepare for the Boston Marathon 2025.

I didn't want to wait, and I didn't want to spend another winter doing lots of long training runs, this time constrained by shorter days and my new habit of only running during daylight.

Step 11
Carb Loading

Apparently, the best carb loading strategy is to add extra carbs to your diet, day by day, during the final three or four days before a marathon.

On day one, about one third of your plate should be carbs! Keep a watch on protein as well. You need adequate protein to maintain and strengthen muscles. The balance of your nutrition should be healthy fruits and vegetables.

I'm sorry that paragraph was so bland! That's me paraphrasing what everybody else says. It really is a struggle to find out what's best, and because we are all "average" and none of us is "average" the "how to" guides are desperately woolly when it comes to explaining the detail on carb loading.

What I need, and what you need could be vastly different, and that will depend on things like age, weight, and general standard of health. And in any case, how big is "one third of a plate"?

My training led to longer distances just before my marathons. Your training might involve tapering in the normal way. Our carb requirements will be different. I entered into the spirit of things, with more rice in my diet, and even some small portions of dessert.

I think we all need personally tailored advice in order to get carb loading right. A running coach or a nutritionist might help us. The professionals may be able to afford that, I can't, so I just had to wing it. As with my calorie counting there's a distinct difference between being conscientious and merely being mindful. Being mindful may not be enough, but it helps us head in the right direction.

Step 12
Visioning

In the last two weeks before the third marathon, I started visioning the way I would handle the course, and I started to imagine my performance. Seven weeks before the event (on the August bank holiday Monday) I had been to Chelmsford to cycle the route. I knew what it was like. Exceedingly rural and simple, lots of minor roads and tracks, some with surfaces that were in desperate need of repair.

Chelmsford Recce
www.dontreadmyblog.com

I knew what the ascents and descents looked like, and I knew some of the "landmarks" along the way. The longest ascent starts as a gentle but unrelenting two kilometres at about 11k. Then a brief respite at 13k, and another long uphill section for a further 3k. In other locations there were short and steep ascents. In all of these places I wanted to maintain a dignified slow jog and "no more walking".

Back home, whether I was training on a mid week short route, or a Sunday long route, I pretended that this was the Chelmsford Marathon. The first 10k, or the last 10k, or (when I was on a 35k run) the major rural section outside the city. Visioning my progress around the Chelmsford course whilst I was running on my familiar London routes.

My training programme is not tapered towards the date of the marathon (cue gasps of astonishment from some seasoned professionals who say you should do reduced distances). On the Sunday just before Chelmsford I covered 35k. The only concession I made to tapering was to forgo my final 10k run on the final Thursday.

The recce of Chelmsford by bike had been worth it. I ran a normal London Bridges 10k training route on the Tuesday, five days before the marathon, and I imagined that I was running the final 10k of the 42k route. In my head I had already mapped the last bit of the Chelmsford 42k onto my 10k route.

At various points in my training runs I was thinking things like; this junction equates to the 37k way point. This stretch is where I have to avoid horse manure. This is the bit where I will struggle through the park, avoiding the toddlers on their tricycles. This corner represents that viaduct. Here's where I have to watch the badly potholed cyclepath with care - no injuries on the final kilometre.

On the final straight I need to spot the photographer, acknowledge the crowd, smile, move my sweat rag away from my race number, thumbs up, smile, finish!

Check my stopwatch. If my pace was right it should say 5 hours 23 minutes. I don't care! I just need to finish. Faster or slower, it doesn't matter. At 61 years of age I will complete my third marathon.

The key message

So this 12 step system is the rudimentary formula that I promised you at the start of this chapter. It includes me eating chocolate sponge cakes. Vision that in your head!

And yes, they were lovely!

Chapter 14 - Plan Your Marathon

Time spent in planning is seldom wasted

All along, I have wanted to be able to run a marathon in less than 5 hours. My training throughout 2023 and 2024 has shown that I should be capable of 5 hours 30 minutes. That would be a personal best. What I had not done before, for any race of any distance, was prepare a documented plan telling me exactly what I was intending to do.

For the Chelmsford Marathon I was going to explore this idea.

Chelmsford Marathon

Based on my later training runs in August and September 2024 my pace sheet had been prepared showing 7 minute 39 second kilometres, and a finish time of 5 hours 22 minutes. Some of my training had clocked a faster pace than that, indicating that I might achieve 5 hours 15 minutes.

Could I try just a little harder? Could I break the 5 hour barrier?

Given the option of trying for 5 hours and failing, or calmy achieving 5 hours 30 minutes, what would you do? I wasn't prepared to risk total retirement from the race. I had trained to secure 5 hours 22 minutes and I wanted to secure just that, 5 hours 22 minutes. Anything better than the 5 hours 52 minutes in Geneva will give me a personal best anyway. In my dreams, I could tag on to the 5 hour pace setter, and do it. But I didn't need to. I just wanted to finish.

The business coach side of me said "plan the work and work the plan". Another one of my mantras! I had planned to do 5 hours 22 minutes, so that was what I was sticking with. I knew the route, I had even tried to memorise the route map, and I had at least memorised the first three waypoints precisely. If any waypoints were off plot or missing (like they were in Milton Keynes) then I could still note my times from my pace sheet and control my early performance.

Run slower!

I had never been better prepared for a marathon. I hadn't come close to total, perfect readiness, but I was happy and confident. The final 18 days of working my secret sauce formula (with the energy gel) were I hoped, just enough to see me accomplish a respectable performance.

However, my long 35k run the week before the marathon had proved that whilst energy gel helped, and delayed the onset of the urge to walk, it only helped me by about 5k. Instead of suffering at around the 25k mark, I reached 30k and then I walked a bit. I yomped the last 5k home. Knowing my history I hastily prepared a new, hybrid plan. Run to the midpoint in 2 hours 30 and yomp the second half in 3 hours. Pretend that the cut off time was 5 hours 30. For Chelmsford it's actually 7 hours. Nonetheless I wanted a good time.

What Could I Have Done Differently?

Muscle strength! Had I learnt more detail about interval training early enough, I would have done it. It was too late in the day to build more robust muscles and glycogen stores. Whilst my calf muscles were big and healthy anyway, I'm sure there was room for them to be bigger and healthier if I tried.

Planning for the Route

In dozens of places I have seen the advice "plan your marathon" and have never fully understood what they mean by that. I took it to mean "plan your race the way you will run it on race day", because none of the advice was explicit about what you actually have to plan for. Particularly when you're doing your first one. How can you plan for something that challenging when you've never done it before?

My early vision of "a plan" was "run one mile" followed by "run one more mile" followed by "run one more mile" etc! Lastly, cross the finish line and "stop running". Surely that's not what they meant?

I think "planning for a wedding" is more in character with what was meant. Start months in advance, work on the venue, the clothing, the transport there and back. Then work out the proceedings for the day. Whether it's a marathon or a wedding, surely there'll be somebody pointing you in the right direction. The process has already been mapped out for you and you simply participate in the day doing what the officials tell you to.

Years in advance I planned my training, which didn't always go to plan! The real marathon planning started approximately two months before the race. By that time I was pretty certain that I was actually going to be ready, and be there running. Seven weeks before Chelmsford I checked the roads, I printed out a map, and I went and cycled around the entire course. That meant that I also did the exact train journey, the way I was going to do it on race day. I found my way from the station to the start line, and then I did a recce of the route, paying particular attention to the quality of the running surface.

In order to try to memorise some of the things that I saw (and wouldn't see again until race day) I gave them a Paddington Bear hard stare in an attempt to imprint them on my brain. There were certain parts of the route like narrow pedestrian bridges, and defective patches of tarmac which I imprinted on that recce. I also attempted to memorise as much of the route map as I could. I took photos of some places, but I prefer to use my imperfect photographic memory rather than the camera on my phone.

Two weeks beforehand, a race day checklist (see Appendix 9) was prepared. I placed an order online for my energy gel sachets. I also started carb loading. I began a daily campaign of checking the weather forecast on the BBC website. Glorious sun it said. Then after a few days, it said almost certain rain on race day. Which then changed again as race day drew closer. Dry and cloudy, then sunny spells. But cold!

Periodically, I would check the route map again. Trying to embed more detail into the picture in my head. I'm lucky I have a bit of photographic memory. Nowhere near photographic like an instamatic camera, but handy nonetheless, as long as I repeatedly work on the images.

One week before, I checked that my kit was complete and serviceable, and I checked that I didn't have to buy anything new. If you're buying new kit, late, then you have to try it out before race day. Never run a marathon wearing anything that you have not already worn on a training run.

My train journey to and from the event was mapped out long beforehand. On the day before the race I bought my paper ticket, going to the station to collect it. I wanted a paper ticket that I could wave at staff if I needed to. And I wanted it in my hand one day early. I didn't want to risk an e-ticket, nor use any technology which might fail on race day.

The afternoon before the race (before the shops closed) I went through my race day checklist and laid out everything for one last check. I bought some chocolate on the Saturday, because I decided I would like to look forward to a little reward immediately after the end of the race.

Running Kit

The night before, I tried on everything I was going to wear or carry while I ran. My fully laden backpack, with water, gel, phone, keys and all the other sundries weighed 4.2kg. I had 19 sachets of gel, which would last 6 hours, and allow me to have one every 20 minutes. My digital watch was on my left wrist, and my pace sheet (in miles) was strapped to my right wrist.

It all felt right, there were no last minute emergencies.

The Memory Game

I looked at the route map again, repeatedly checking and looking away, to test my powers of recall. I was determined to memorise with pinpoint accuracy where those first three waypoints were. Mile One, the far end of Admirals Park at the treeline, the precise point where the path crosses an expanse of grass and goes into the trees. Mile Two, just after the Kiddi Caru Day Nursery access road, just before the junction of Fox Burrows Lane and Lordship Lane (Anglia Ruskin University Writtle Campus). Mile Three, the far end of the Sturgeons Farm complex at the entrance to the old farmhouse, just before the bridlepath ends. Whether these first three waypoints had signs or not, I knew the locations and I could check my time against my pace sheet.

Not only that, I noted that there was a narrow pedestrian bridge in Admirals Park just half a mile away from the start. I had struggled to work out how big the entry list might be. Various "running calendar" websites showed it as 4,000 or 1,500 or 1,000. The official website, and the race pack from the organisers didn't give a figure at all. I had to assume that 1,000 runners would all be turning up at the same time to cross that bridge! My strategy? Take no risks, go with the flow, slow, fast, or whatever.

Mainly, I need to keep to my pace according to my pace sheet. There's another narrow bridge soon after Mile One followed immediately by a sharp left 90° turn where one third of the cyclepath is impassable due to overgrown shrubs. Same again, take no risks. At least these places should be less congested on the return leg.

The course on *plotaroute* can be expanded, and it gives more detail on elevation.

Chelmsford Marathon
www.plotaroute.com/route/2286466

The longest uphill stretch was a bit of decent rural road from 10.7k to 12.5k. It's early in the race, and I should be able to maintain my pace with no issues. The steepest hill is 4.4% at 16.1k. Right outside Dukes Farm. When I cycled that it was a first gear hill, but I didn't find it worrisome. The corresponding bit at the far end of the loop is further west, going up Millers Green Road at around 19k. That may be less than 4.4% but that's the section which I flagged up as the most troubling. I hoped to keep up a slow jog, and because it's OK to not be OK, I imagined walking to the summit and regaining lost time on later downhill bits.

I also knew that I would have to go through a housing estate in Roxwell at about the 10k mark, where the road surface is low quality and there are cars parked along each side of the road. At 26k there's a gentle uphill stretch with a less than gentle perfume as you pass some exceedingly smelly cow sheds! I said to myself that I would adjust my pace as required, being mindful of my pace sheet, but slowing down if there was any danger, and speeding up (a little) to minimise the time spent inhaling unwelcome smells!

Temperature

The forecast said that the day before the marathon would have rain, and that it would be dry on race day. Hence I expected some surface water and I was determined to avoid all of it. Race day was going to have a chilly 5°C start with lots of sunshine, and the temperature would rise to 10° by mid afternoon. It would cloud over progressively as the day went on.

That's fine! Definitely cool at the start, and ideal temperatures at the end. I went back to refer to my records. The log told me that over the past ten years I had run wearing tracksuit trousers at temperatures of 0° and below, and I had run in shorts at 2° and above. Clearly, I would be wearing shorts! As a precaution I would also carry my tracksuit trousers stuffed into the backpack. That left my options open. Winds were forecast to be gentle, at around 4 to 7mph. If for any reason it became colder and/or especially windy, I was prepared to stop and put on the tracksuit trousers. I was hoping that I wouldn't need to.

This was the level of detail I went into with my planning. It was more of a plan than I had ever established before.

Chapter 15 - Marathon 3 Chelmsford

Sunday 13 Oct 2024

As usual, I was up early. I put on my exact running kit for the race, and I went outside at 6.00am. The temperature in London was 6° C. The BBC website said that the temperature in Chelmsford was lower, but it would be 6° by 9.00am and it would rise to 10° later in the day. What I wanted to know was whether I had selected the right level of clothing. Yes! Exactly right, at 6° my legs felt OK, my double layer top was appropriate, and if I ran like this then my legs would be warm enough. Wearing any more layers of clothing would have made things a little too warm for me.

And these days, now that I understood the importance of carb loading, I had some breakfast. A Japanese breakfast of rice, *miso shiru* (vegetables in a bean paste broth) and a large helping of grapes. And more than one cup of tea! I also prepared a flask of tea, a cheese and pickle sandwich, an apple, a banana and a small chocolate bar to take with me. That would be my picnic lunch in the park at the end of the race. Along with a complete change of clothes I crammed all of this into my usual drop bag and I made a mental note to have a bigger bag next time!

Dressed for the race, I then strapped the pace sheet to my right wrist. It was in miles. A bunch of unfamiliar numbers showing 11 minute 27 miles! At least for the first half, and then 13 minute 08 miles for the remainder. Optimistically, it had a finish time of 5 hours and 23 minutes. The idea was that I was going to stick with the 5 hour pace setter (assuming there was one) for the first half of the race, and then adjust to my yomping pattern for the second half. What I really wanted was to beat 5 hours 30.

Although my hybrid pace sheet showed everything in miles my brain still planned the yomping in kilometres. For marathon organisers reading this book, please prepare a second set of waypoints in kilometres! Please!

Wearing waterproof clothing over my running kit, I boarded the 0726 train at Liverpool Street Station. There wasn't any rain, but I had prepared some cheap overalls in any case, for warmth. I could discard them at the start and let the charity shop workers take them.

Chelmsford is a small city, and their marathon is a low key affair which doesn't get headline billing like many others. The online information and the PDF race guide aren't as extensive as others, and I struggled to work out how big the entry list might be. Anything from 1,000 to 4,000 from what I could see. The cut off time also varied depending on which website you looked at. At least the official home page made the cut off clear, it was 7 hours. That allowed me the luxury of a bit of leeway if anything failed to go to plan during the race.

The event village in Central Park was small, and well staffed by volunteers. A fair amount of sunshine did its best to take the chill off the morning. The dappled sunshine made the autumn colours on the trees look wonderful, but it didn't do anything to improve the temperature around the start.

Both the marathon and half marathon take place concurrently with the *half* starting 30 minutes after the main race. The races share the same course until roughly the 10k mark. I asked about the numbers and about pace setters. There were more than 1,000 entries for the *half*, and more than 500 for the marathon. Wow, that is small! Blue bibs up to 500+ for us, and (for half marathoners) red bibs numbered from 1,000 onwards

There were pace setters, but the arrangement was informal. Rather than sporting colourful pennants from a backpack, they wore a second bib on their back.

As we prepared for the start I saw one runner with number 535 on his bib so I assumed that "about 550" was a fair guess for the number of runners. I later learnt that some had deferred to next year, and that just 387 people were due to run the marathon. I dropped my bag at the big tent, gave my overalls to a charity stall in the event village, and I went off to perform my stretches routine.

Just before the start I took the first of the 19 energy sachets I'd brought with me. That left me with one to be consumed every 20 minutes, and a couple of spares if I needed them.

The starting pens were labelled from 1 hour 30 through to 2 hours 45 and that was it. They were the half marathon times. There were no signs for the full marathon so I just went to the back of the pack. A few minutes before the 9.00am start, as I was taking out my phone to call my wife, I spotted two pace setters, both with 5 hour 30 bibs. I didn't have time to chat to them before the race, and I didn't spot any other pace setters near the start line.

I had just finished my phone call, put on my thin lightweight gloves, and we were off.

I passed over the start line rather quickly compared to any of my other races, just 90 seconds after the gun, and as far as I could make out I was the last runner to set off. That gained me a special mention over the public address system! I knew that the cyclepath at the start was in poor condition, although because I wasn't boxed in by other runners I could see where I was going, and I was able to cautiously check the placement of my feet. Luxury! Well "luxury" in the sense that I could *see* the dodgy running surface!

Round the weird cyclepath roundabout at 50m, under the viaduct, and off on the meandering path through Central Park and then Admirals Park. I missed the official photographer at the roundabout as he was adjusting his camera after trying to capture the first 500 runners!

It didn't take long before I caught up with the 5 hour 30 pace setters. They had acquired a "bus" of about eight runners. Checking our pace sheets we were all ahead of schedule, and that allowed me a time to indulge in a short chat. They told me that there *was* a 5 hour pace setter, and his name was Rob. Then I moved ahead of them, tried to adjust my pace to match my intended 11 minute 27 second miles, and I assumed that sooner or later I would find Rob.

At the Mile One waypoint I was about 60 seconds ahead of schedule. I eased off a little more. According to plan I took one energy gel sachet at 20 minutes.

Before reaching Mile Two I met Andrew from Maidstone Harriers. He was the 5 hour 15 pace setter though he had nobody in his "bus". I wondered if I should stay with him, but I was mindful of my plan to do a faster first half and a slower second half. We talked briefly and he told me that the course was longer than a proper marathon, it wasn't in accordance with "IAAF" standards, and that although it was "only a little longer" he was fairly sure he would cross the line on time at 5 hours 15. I failed to ask what "a little longer" meant. Five metres? Fifty metres?

The sky had clouded over, and I was glad to have my lightweight gloves. At Mile Two I was still ahead of my schedule by about 60 seconds. I had actually run that mile at my exact pace, but I was ahead of schedule because I had built in a buffer from my first mile. It was the same when I reached the Mile Three waypoint. I still hadn't caught up with Rob, because (I assumed) that his pace matched mine perfectly, and we were maintaining a uniform separation between us. As we left the cyclepath and joined a proper road there was another official photographer. I was unprepared for that photo opportunity, and hoped it would come out OK.

Now the undulations started. And the road surface was a mix of good and bad. My cycle recce had prepared me for this, and I ran a few uneventful miles up to the Mile Six waypoint at Roxwell. However, some faster runners started passing me at quite a pace. By the time the fourth or fifth one zoomed passed me, wearing flimsy clothing with no backpacks nor water, I realised that these were the leaders of the half marathon. That was a new experience. Being overtaken by Speedy Gonzalez after only a "short" distance.

By Mile Six my buffer had increased a little, to 90 seconds. I was running faster than I wanted to, but that was OK because I had a long ascent coming up very soon. I was still on track with consuming one energy gel sachet every 20 minutes, though I wasn't getting any sort of mental buzz doing that. I reminded myself of the science behind it, and that although I could feel nothing right now, I would probably benefit later in the race.

It wasn't until Roxwell that we encountered spectators. Nice friendly people and applause and exhortations. And I adopted my typical banter, exchanging words with some of them "that's a lovely smile" and "you're my friend". On one street corner in Roxwell the four noisy little ones who shouted at me deserved a special response "wow, my fan club, thanks for coming out to cheer me on".

In Roxwell the course split with the *half* going off to the south as we went north. I also picked up a companion for about 800m. We chatted intermittently, he was also doing his third marathon. He had done 5 hrs 18 mins on his first, and 4 hrs 40 mins on his second. Confiding in me that he has no idea how he achieved a sub 5 hour finish the second time around.

I mentioned my cycle recce, and that the tough ascent was just ahead. Two kilometres of gentle and solid uphill from 11 to 13k, then a brief respite for a bit, followed by another 2k of ascent after that. I wasn't going to be able to match his pace going uphill, and I bid him good luck as he went ahead of me. I had remembered all of the route detail from my race plan, but what I hadn't taken account of was the continuation (beyond 15k) of even more and more relentless uphill, on the way to the hamlet of Birds Green beyond Willingale. It's a very long gentle uphill stretch, I had cycled it without much trouble. But trying to run it is a completely different ball game! I had forgotten my research which told me that the steepest hill at 16k had a 4.4% gradient.

Naismith's

Somewhere on the long ascent from 11k to 16k I passed a group of hikers heading in the same direction, and all wearing heavy backpacks with large dayglo green covers. They might have been older Boy Scouts or a Duke of Edinburgh group. If nothing else it took my mind off the current distraction of my own troubling uphill journey, as I pondered theirs. It also brought back a long lost memory of a time when I went hiking in the Derbyshire Dales.

When I lived in Nottingham (in my late twenties) an informal group at the office had decided that one weekend we should go hiking in the Dales. That introduced me to the Naismith's rule. Part way around this marathon course

> I now remembered that such a rule existed, but I couldn't remember the precise detail! William Naismith was a Scottish mountaineer who established a rule of thumb in 1892. Allow one hour for every 5 kilometres horizontally and add one hour for every 600 metres vertically (whether up or down).
>
> Wracking my brain (for those elusive numbers) kept me occupied for two or three minutes, though nothing came of it. Even if I'd remembered the formula I had no current way of knowing what the elevation of this course was. Over the preceding weeks I had examined the course profile online a few times, but I hadn't been inclined to memorise 50 or so separate bits of up and down.
>
> That's probably just as well. Although my mental arithmetic is generally good, I don't think I could have added any more value to my race by having precise figures right now. I carried on, thinking that "this is a good thing", because knowing the numbers might have been counterproductive!
>
> What it might mean, for future events, is that the Naismith's rule could enable me to adjust my expectations by converting my pace on a level route, to an overall pace for a hilly route.

It was a struggle to keep running. By the time I reached the Mile Ten waypoint I reasoned that some walking was permissible. I checked my watch and my pace sheet, and I was a mere six seconds behind schedule. I had use up the buffer zone I had previously built up and I said to myself "you know what, 10 miles, that's 16k, and if I've done 16k and matched my target, I can ease off briefly, I've deserved it"!

Mindful of my own philosophy "it's OK to not be OK" and self taught on the subject energy consumption, I reasoned that "the precursor" of "hitting the wall" would arrive sooner if I continued to battle uphill like this. Nowhere near proper fatigue, but achy calf muscles that were unaccustomed to ascents of this nature. Knowing that the two solutions are "stop and rest" or "slow down drastically" I decided to slow down a little and adopt a power walk, rather than continue to jog uphill. I yomped! I yomped the remaining uphill stretch to the T junction by Tile House Farm at Birds Green. And I expected to run from there.

Rounding that corner, exchanging pleasantries with the marshals, I started running again. I reach the Mile 11 waypoint and promptly started walking again. I had also wearied of taking one gel sachet every 20 minutes, and I decided to scale back on that, to take one only when it felt right. Oh dear, what about my plan? I was adrift on two counts, I was supposed to run to the half way stage, and only resort to yomping for the second half, and I was supposed to consume gel routinely every 20 minutes. To improve my mindset I adopted a variation of my classic yomping. Rather than doing the walk 2 run 2 pattern which I've used regularly in the past I was aiming for an improved ratio, walk 2 run 3, or even better. One flight plan, one million in flight adjustments!

It started at Mile 11. I walked for two telegraph poles, and ran for four. And I repeated that for a few minutes until the course turned left over the River Roding and up towards Millers Green. Then the telegraph poles vanished! This was the worst hill from my cycle recce. Not the steepest gradient on the course (I had passed that already), but this was the hill that caused me the most trouble by bike. A tiny rural road with random plant life erupting in vibrant shades of green along the centre line of the road. A centre line which was completely unmolested by tyres because the narrow road confined cars to a strictly limited amount of tarmac. As I climbed to the top of the hill some running took place, a lot of walking took place, and I had some pleasant chats with the marshals that I passed. This race had more marshals, first aid posts, and water stations than any other I had done.

With the Millers Green hill behind me I was back to my classic yomping, using my improved ratio, and I managed a half decent pace as far as the foot of the hill by the sewage works at Willingale. I passed that and then the ascent started. Water was cascading down the hill. Yes, it had rained the previous evening, but I hadn't expected this much surface water. Avoiding the worst of it, I went up the hill, sticking to the centre line of the road where the camber is better, sometimes to the right, sometimes to the left, giving way to the four cars which travelled the hill at the same time as I did. The toes of my left foot momentarily became damp. I detest running with wet feet. I immediately adjusted course. Fortunately the damp was trivial and short lived.

The village of Willingale came into view at the top of the hill, and so did the burst water main in the centre of the road!

Just beyond Willingale the course looped around on itself for about five miles. That meant that a lot of marshals and spectators had gathered at the mid point. As I passed the junction many of the faster runners were joining the loop for the second time, they were miles ahead of me! There were still a reasonable number of us starting our first loop. I was adjusting to a welcome section of slightly more level road, and I adopted a more regulated process of yomping. Taking off my gloves I called my wife to let her know that I'd reached the half way stage at 2 hrs 36 mins. Six minutes behind schedule, but nothing alarming.

The slower time meant that I had to revise my plan for the second half, I also had to factor in a bit more fatigue due to the hills. This was the same as last time! And the time before that! Getting to roughly the half way stage of a marathon and discovering that I am not good and predicting my performance on the day. This time I blamed the hills, when I really should have been blaming myself. On the plus side (and for a short time) I needed my baseball cap to keep the sun out of my eyes. My gloves were no longer needed. The sunshine was intermittent, and coincided with much of the five mile loop to the south east of Willingale.

Should I now resume my energy gel strategy? Taking one sachet every 20 minutes? And hope that this would reinvigorate my motivation to run? Whilst my stomach was not overloaded in any way, it was telling me that the situation was not normal. I resolved to stick with my newly developed "take one when you feel like it" strategy, and in the end I didn't use any energy gel after the half way mark.

Soon after Mile 15, looping back up towards Willingale, there's a gentle ascent. That's the section where Andrew caught up with me and continued on. He was now accompanied, bringing the total of his 5 hour 15 bus to him plus one. There were a number of runners ahead of me and behind, and a bit more motor traffic than I'd expected. One or two foolish drivers, and a lot of careful ones.

As we approached Spains Hall Farm an enormous modern tractor was heading towards us. He kindly pulled over to let a small group pass without them having to alter course, and then he slowly crawled past me, giving me adequate space to use my bit of the road. Spains Hall Farm was devoid of smelly cows. Thankfully!

Somewhere between Mile 16 and Mile 17 I was passed by the 5 hour 30 pace setters. Clearly my pace was not where it should have been! I was not going to beat 5 hours 30. This was all too familiar from my earlier marathons. I needed to put in some more effort. By the time I reached Mile 19 I was back to my run 2 walk 2 system. But I wasn't doing that consistently. Not only that, there were no other runners in sight. I was now alone.

Although the later stages of the course are nowhere near as hilly as the earlier ones, there were a few ascents. Quite a lot actually. My brain started playing tricks on me. I knew that the last 12k had more descents than ascents, but it didn't feel like that. The same thing had happened to me one year earlier on the Tonbridge Half Marathon. If I was on the level, or on a gentle descent, my body was convinced that I was still running uphill. My classic yomping was taking a hit, because I walked, especially on the authentic ascents. I still maintained the run 2 walk 2 system as much as I could, but the overall ratio was falling below where it ought to have been.

Could I simply power walk the remainder of the course? I did the mental arithmetic, if I started power walking now, I wouldn't reach the finish line until

6 hours 14. A long way off my target, better than Milton Keynes, but worse than Geneva. My legs weren't playing along. I couldn't maintain the pace of my usual power walk. I tried. I also tried extended sections of running, and I was still caving in to muscle fatigue after every few hundred metres. At least I had a 7 hour cut off to help me. If I had to walk at a purposeful pace (one step down from my power walk) I could still finish before the sweeper bus. But I was convinced I could do better than that.

Somewhere on the backroads I encountered a fire engine. Off to my distant left, twos and blues going. At the top of the hill it turned towards me, filling the entire width of the road, coming down the hill at a purposeful speed. The driver saw me, and lifted his foot off the accelerator. The engine note changed. By which time I had already decided to completely move off the road. I signalled him to pass me as I stepped up onto a decent bit of grass verge. It was the only time during the entire marathon that I actually stopped and stood still. The driver and I both smiled knowingly as we passed.

Clearly I was now one of the very tail enders. The marshals were still there at every key road junction, they were kind, and by this stage both they and I were more talkative. In truth we were alleviating the boredom. I sang "sunshine came softly through my, through my window today" and later asked some marshals where the sun had gone. I put my gloves on again. My new tune became "what a day for a daydream" as I tried to keep my mind off muscle fatigue. Then at the next marshal I resorted to humour:

"Can you help me with a recommendation?"
Puzzled, the marshal responded "a recommendation for what?"
"A psychiatrist!"

Cue laughter all round. The timing and the delivery of that one had been perfect, almost as if we had rehearsed it.

It was so funny that the tame ducks in the grounds of Newney House joined in with the laughter:

"wak wak wak wak wak-wak-wak"

And that set off the wild ducks on the other side of the road:

"wak wak wak wak wak-wak-wak"

I marvelled at my ability to entertain ducks! I was heading up yet another gentle ascent towards Cow Watering Campus, and that would be followed by the final three miles along the cyclepath towards the centre of Chelmsford. Whilst I'd been walking (a little too often) I had been formulating a revised, revised plan. Another of my one million in flight adjustments! I was going to do my best to run the final three miles, on the dodgy cyclepaths, because I knew that the last three miles were level. As I passed Mile 23 my arithmetic told me that if I did *not* run, I was on for 6 hours 10.

I began running again, and I caught and passed two tail enders. Slowing briefly, to let them know that a walk to the end would lead them to a 6 hour 10 finish, that I was now trying to hit 6 hours, and that meant a constant steady jog. Fordy (his name was Paul, but it said "Fordy" on the back of his shirt) joined me briefly at a jogging pace. He and I had passed each other a handful of times throughout the course, each time having a very brief chat. By the time I reached Mile 24 I was on my own again. I slowed to a power walk two or three times, but I kept up a meaningful jog as often as I could.

As I reached Mile 25 I checked my watch. Not good! Six hours is possible, but it's going to take a considerable effort! Luckily, Admirals Park and Central Park were not as busy as I'd feared. The kids were no problem, the dog walkers were doing their best to give me a clear passage, but a couple of the dogs had no idea about the etiquette of running. Narrowly avoiding two collisions I was looking ahead trying to spot the Mile 26 waypoint. Surely I should be there by now, and I should also be able to see the viaduct? How much longer do I have to do this?

Another check of the watch. The bit from Mile 25 to Mile 26 was the longest mile I've ever run. I was borderline on target for exactly 6 hours. Passing Mile 26 I could see the viaduct. I could also see that my route was largely clear of people. I ran faster. I felt like I was doing my 6 min 30 per kilometre pace.

I could see and hear the finish line. It seemed really far away! I know what it's like getting from 42k to 42.195k. But getting from Mile 26 to the finish line was *what* in yards? I had no idea! It just felt like an awfully long way to me.

As I passed under the viaduct, going left a little, my stopwatch said 5 hrs 59 mins 30 secs. I could see the weird little roundabout. I picked up the pace even more, my 6 minute per kilometre pace, the family with the baby buggy were startled, tail enders don't normally run this fast do they? The family moved out of the way just in time, I reached the roundabout, 10 seconds remained, I sprinted for all I was worth, taking the straightest line I could through the curve, and powering on to the finish line. Simultaneously I smiled for the photographer, pressed the button on my stopwatch and checked. My watch said 6 hrs 00 mins 15 secs.

For Chelmsford I had been far better educated, better prepared, equipped with energy gel, weighed far less than I had for any other race I'd done, and I had been visioning everything I was going to experience. It still wasn't enough to get the time I wanted. However, I wasn't last! John Backley would have been happy that I finished ahead of seven other runners. But I was disappointed. Mainly because my mental arithmetic had failed me. My number crunching before Mile 23 (just before I resumed running) had led me to believe that I could achieve a sub 6 hour finish. I had missed that revised, revised target by 15 seconds.

I could claim that there were any number of reasons why my performance on the day was less than I had hoped for. It was cold, the surfaces were sub standard, the ascents were much more than I was used to, and I had not had enough time to perfect the right energy gel strategy. But the simple fact was that I was under prepared all round, I lacked calf muscle strength, and my metabolism of energy gel is nothing like the average discussed in the science materials. I could certainly do with a lot more muscle in my legs. Some weight training in addition to the running might have helped.

Added to that, in the year since the Tonbridge Half Marathon, I had experienced many more injuries than normal, and I had been through extended periods with no training runs. Having registered for marathons in April 2024, in September 2024, and in October 2024, I withdrew my entries for the first two due to the lengthy breaks interfering with my training.

The main reason for my commitment to the October 2024 race was that I wanted to do this whilst I was still 61 years old, and not to have to spend another six months training through the winter (with limited daylight hours) before the Boston Marathon in April 2025. Secondly, I was also fit and injury free in mid October 2024. Perhaps not in perfect condition, but given the recent, rocky twelve month history, I wanted to seize the moment and run. There was no certainty that I would remain injury free for the "next one".

After the race, the Chelmsford results were published online very quickly. I had an email on my phone within 90 minutes. I was on the train home at the time, and I had a look. My chip time was 6 hrs 00 mins 14 secs. I scrolled through the results, and as he had predicted, Andrew (the pace setter) had finished exactly as he wanted, a few seconds ahead of 5 hrs 15 mins. Hang on! Didn't he say the course was longer than the regular marathon distance?

Once I was back home, I checked. Nothing on the Chelmsford Marathon website nor in the PDF race guides mention the "IAAF" standards. Neither was there any mention anywhere of the actual distance. *Plotaroute* says that the course was 42.544k and not the standard 42.195k. That's an extra 349 metres!

That's why Mile 26 to the finish line seemed so far!

I reasoned that the route must have been prepared to fit the natural layout of the local roads, and the IAAF requirements came in a poor second to the practicality of getting things done. The start/finish line could have been moved. But that would have placed it in a really awkward location, blocking the busy pedestrian bridge over the River Can right next to the viaduct.

So I did some calculations. I established that if I had been timed over 42.195k I would have completed the race in 5 hrs 57 mins 18 secs. My mental arithmetic had been right all along. I was not quite so disappointed after all!

Weird isn't it? In Milton Keynes, I had done an extra 600m. In Chelmsford, an extra 349m. It was only in Geneva that I actually did the correct distance!

In a more general sense have I achieved what I set out to do? Undoubtedly yes! I wanted to lose some weight. Over the past twenty years my body mass has gone down an astonishing 24%. I wanted to complete a marathon. During that time I have completed *three* marathons. My younger self had clearly done something right. Changing course in my mid forties had made all the difference.

And so far I'm doing well on this score . . .

> *The objective is to live longer not to kill yourself.*

The third marathon was not exactly the experience that I had hoped for. I now realise that some of us are not really cut out to be marathon runners.

Perhaps I should take up chucking spears?

Or more realistically, my distance is 10k and maybe I should just stick to that?

Chapter 16 - The Future

The Power of Imagination

Imagine a future you. When you retire, where will you live? Who will be living with you? What will your daily life look like? And your special occasions? How and when, will you spend time with your friends and relatives? Do you have grandchildren who come to visit?

This is an exercise which I work over in my mind from time to time. Especially the bit involving really old age. End of life stuff! How will I cope when I'm extremely old? What will my physical health, and my mental health be like? Will I be able to live independently and still walk to the shops? Will I be in a care home?

A day in the life of ninety something Paul, will see me living in my own home, in the centre of a large city, where I can walk to the supermarket, the bank, and the Post Office. Where I can walk to a restaurant or two, or a pub or two. Where I can live a normal life, for as long as possible. If that means that I will be living in the centre of London, or Geneva, or Tokyo, then I will also have to be fit enough to use public transport. A day in the life of a ninety something Paul will start early, perhaps not as early as 5.00am the way that it does now, but it will involve daily exercise.

I don't do *Rajio Taiso* (pronounced "rah-jee-o tie so", meaning Radio Exercise) but instead I prefer my own unique circuit training style workout which is based on my school day PE lessons, and the stretches I outlined in Chapter 5. When I'm older I might adopt *Rajio Taiso* instead. This link to a 3 minute video gives you some idea of what *Rajio Taiso* looks like. On some Japanese TV stations, variations of this sort of routine are broadcast every morning of the week.

Rajio Taiso
www.youtube.com

When it comes to ninety something Paul, early mornings will start with a routine of gentle stretches and floor exercises. Then a brisk walk to the supermarket and back. Breakfast with my wife. A leisurely morning of reading "the newspapers". A light lunch. An afternoon walk in the park, or possibly a visit to something interesting for mental and cultural stimulation. A simple dinner at home, or out, or with friends, or with the grandchildren coming to visit. My late afternoons and evenings will be filled with reading and writing. Monthly "event days" will see us, as a couple, visiting theatres, or exhibitions, or other extravaganza. I will give up foreign holidays and flying. And wherever I live, I will have a holiday once a year, without leaving the country.

I have a dozen ideas for books. All non fiction. Over the years, work has started on a number of them and then they've been quietly side lined. Several more books are nothing more than ambitious ideas which have yet to even germinate.

I will never truly retire. I will be semi-retired until the day I die, the author, the public speaker, the old fella with a dash of eccentricity, who has retained a remarkable fitness, because he's rather obsessed with healthy eating and proper exercise.

There will still be the visit, in March and in September each year, to the 400m track for me to monitor my performance. Even if I have to take the bus there and back. And you? What does your future hold? Is there a plan?

Does it involve another marathon? Don't rule it out! Back in 2011, when he was 100 years old, Londoner Fauja Singh finished the Toronto Marathon in 8 hrs 25 mins 18 secs, ahead of five other competitors.

Fauja Singh
www.youtube.com

Toronto was his eighth marathon! He did his first when he was 89 years old!

Another Marathon

Here's an expression I've seen a number of times, in a number of places. It crops up in various business coaching materials, but with no precise attribution. I believe this is an old military adage:

"Time spent in planning is seldom wasted."

It's important to note that having a *goal* is not the same thing as having a *plan*. Looking back at my running history since 2005, clearly all I had was a goal, or a dream. As my own business coach once said to me "that's not so much a dream, but a complete hallucination"! Anyway, it was a starting point.

What really matters is using the goal to build an implementation plan, and to turn the dream into a reality. As Peter Drucker said:

"Implementation is everything."

In a haphazard way, my ideas took years to evolve into something that you might call a plan. It was not committed to writing at the start. Nor has it ever been one single document setting out a neat timeline, and proper milestones along the way. It wasn't like that, because it wasn't supposed to be a *business* plan.

What evolved was a collection of documents. Spreadsheets for logging progress. Some Word docs for maintaining a "runner's diary", allowing me to capture a lot more detail than the "notes" column in a spreadsheet. But the most valuable and flexible bit of the plan has been the personal wiki with its built in search facility.

That's where I've been able to add extensive notes about things like health and fitness reports on the web, about forthcoming races, and other links to useful resources. The wiki also hosts my "injury log" as it's a lot easier to search one wiki than it is to search twenty spreadsheets over twenty years.

The most rudimentary part of the plan has been the maintenance of the running log on the spreadsheets. The records of dates, distances and times. And weight, and blood pressure. All the other bits have developed from those fundamentals.

Does it all point to another marathon? Yes and no! Let's first consider the three that I've already done. What characterises them?

Number 1 - Milton Keynes - 6 hours, 28 minutes and 24 seconds.

I was ready I thought, in terms of stamina and running ability. I was mentally prepared, and I was confident that I could complete the distance. Yet I was woefully under educated and I lacked a plan for each stage of the race. Excess water intake, and a completely uncoordinated adventure consuming energy gel, upset what little strategy I had, and that caused my downfall.

Number 2 - Geneva - 5 hours, 52 minutes and 31 seconds.

A stupid mistake could have been avoided. I could probably have finished at around the 5 hour mark, maybe more, maybe less. Forgetting to put sun block on my legs, and suffering both sun burn and aching muscles probably added an extra hour to the time I could have achieved.

Number 3 - Chelmsford - 5 hours, 57 minutes and 18 seconds.

Nothing more, and nothing less than "satisfactory". This was looking good, with a wide ranging plan, and a vastly improved knowledge of health and fitness. It was a calm, measured approach, with a plan that should have led to an improved time. I did a lot of study and explored a good deal of science, but there is no substitute for training on the actual type of terrain that matches the course. Running on hilly routes means that training on level routes is not enough.

The Trend

Back in Chapter 6 I said "the older I get, the faster I get! That's a trend that can't last?" Well that was true. With the knowledge I now have, and with fewer injury breaks, and more time to train, I might be able to do better. But then again, I'm an old man now!

So you never know, I might just keep on keeping on, because that's been the pattern so far. Every year I will enter the ballot for the London Marathon and see what happens. Whether I do London or not, I will keep running. And I will almost certainly do some official 10k races.

And you? What does your future hold? Is there a plan?

Retrospective

Since about the age of eight, when I first started winning races in the swimming gala at school, my physical education has been defined by the teachers who encouraged my swimming prowess. When I was 18 years old I qualified as a lifeguard, having joined a training program which was being run at the pool next door to my school. I was a keen learner, and I was good at remembering everything the instructors taught me. In the end, I only ever worked as a lifeguard for one summer, at a different pool.

And you don't eat before a long swim! I have carried that knowledge with me forever, and I had imported it (wisely I thought) into my running hobby. That's why I didn't eat before major races. It works for anything less than two hours. It does not work when you're running longer distances!

Technically, the dream to "complete a marathon" was fulfilled when I did the first one in Milton Keynes in 2013. With a bit more persistency and consistency I might still be able to secure that sub 5 hour marathon which I've always wanted. However, a win is a win. Any experienced football team will tell you, as will any experienced solicitor, that a messy win is still a win.

Then again, I'm not a young man. I wasn't a young man when I started this! What I've shown is that even somebody like me can complete a marathon. I've shown the pain, the heartache and the anguish. And I've shown that keeping a positive mental attitude has seen me through all of this, even when my ability has fallen short.

The "how to" guides troubled me a lot, and so has the mainstream media with the way that they portray marathons. I was under the misapprehension that anybody with a bit of drive can do this.

Perhaps I've criticised them more than they deserved. It imagine that it's not that easy to compile a "one size fits all" guide, or a news report, or some entertaining TV coverage. Instead, what I've tried to do is tell the true story of one man's journey. A journey that has become more ordered and more well defined as each year passes. And a journey which has required more time and effort studying, than actually running! I've tried to create an ordered system.

The alternative is chaos. Remember the bit where I described a scene from *The Day of the Triffids*? David's foraging had caused the decayed infrastructure of London to collapse around him, returning man made structures to nature. That's entropy. That's the second law of thermodynamics. It's all about order and chaos. Without a conscientious effort on our part to instil order the way that we humans see it, nature will instil order the way that nature sees it. We might think of it as chaos. However, nature may think that tangled weeds and undergrowth are the natural order of things.

Likewise, without a conscientious effort on our part to instil order on the capitalist excesses of our modern lives, we could all just vegetate on the couch in front of a screen, and live off ultra processed food delivered by couriers to our doorsteps. Instilling order is what Canguilhem was talking about when he said:

"Health is threat management, and the ability to adapt to one's environment."

All I have to do now is continue the daily campaign of threat management, and continue to adapt to the ever changing circumstances of modern life. I've established a healthy life style, that's the biggest difference between forty something Paul and sixty something Paul. I've created my own positive, self reinforcing feedback loop. Healthy living leads to more healthy living.

For now, I look forward to seeing you at some undisclosed date in the future, alongside me, on the London Marathon. In the meantime you can find me and a whole bunch of other people like me, by following #runnersofmastodon.

@proactivepaul
www.mastodon.social

Chapter 17 - A Letter to my Younger Self

Older and Wiser

I don't yet know what the ultimate *end of the story* looks like, but I wanted to show you the way that it looks right now, and I can do that best by sharing with you a letter which a sixty something Paul might write to a forty something Paul.

Dear Mid Forties Paul

Run slower!

When you're out practising, you will see some old men, doing a preposterously slow and steady run. And they can do that ad infinitum. That's what you're aiming for. It's all about endurance, it's not about speed, and it's not really about distance. It's about stamina! Being able to run like that for hours on end. Aim to maintain the same pace throughout.

It's a false economy to start off a bit faster and to "bank" some spare minutes as a notional safety net. It never works out like that. A fast first half and a slow second half risk a worse performance overall. The fatigue mounts up sooner, and hits you harder in the second half. Keep it slow and steady from start to finish. There will be some trial and error, but you will find the right pace as you train. A stopwatch on one wrist and a pace sheet on the other are what you need.

There is a world of difference in the strategies for doing short distance and long distance running. Humans are not designed to run for hours on end. When your long runs last more than two hours you have to use energy supplements. Study a little about glycogen and fat. Under pressure, fat alone does not metabolise quickly enough to allow you to maintain a fast pace. After two hours the glycogen supplies soon vanish.

You need to plan to maintain the body's access to readily available glycogen. Otherwise, you might hit the wall, or more likely you will hit the precursor to hitting the wall. Your body will conserve energy by automatically adjusting to a pitifully slow walking pace! Bigger, stronger calf muscle will help, both in terms of sheer performance and with larger energy stores. That's why interval training is recommended. A wise approach to energy management will help you stay in control.

Adopt a holistic attitude to health and fitness, because *health* and *fitness* go hand in hand. Weight management is the key to good health. What matters most is *what* you eat. It matters more than your exercise routine. Dr Giles Yeo says "you cannot outrun a bad diet". In his dialogue he goes on to say:

"The only way to gain weight is to eat more than you burn, and the only way to lose weight is to burn more than you eat. It is a fundamental law of physics, and there is no way of getting around it."

Log everything. Use the metric system. Log your time, distance, pace, weight, and blood pressure. And regularly write some notes in a "runners diary". Keep a food diary when necessary, keep a calorie count sometimes, and always keep an injury log. As the years pass, these are some of the most valuable documents which you will refer to time and time again.

If you don't measure it you don't manage it!

Find your own routine, your own style, your own pace. Don't try to fit in with others unless their target pace is a perfect match for your target pace. Once you know what works for you, keep at it. Keep on keeping on!

Your achievements will stack up. And eventually plateau. All that means is that you've found your optimum. You cannot repeatedly reduce your weight and you cannot repeatedly increase your performance forever.

And then when you become really old, things will gradually decline. That's normal. In order to maintain a clear picture always do the RAF fitness test every March and every September. Time yourself over six laps of a 400m track. Log it. You start by aiming to be better than your younger self. Then you're aiming to regulate a gradual, managed decline into old age. The objective is to live longer not to kill yourself.

You have the physical strength, and the mental capacity, to do everything you want to. You are perfectly capable of living a long, fit, healthy and happy life. And I wish you all the best.

Yours sincerely

Paul.

Mid Sixties Paul

Appendix 1 - My Why What How

Chapter One asked you to grab a pen and a sheet of paper, and write down the answers to these questions:

1. How did you get here?
2. How did you end up reading this book about running?
3. Why?
4. What are you hoping to achieve?
5. Where does it all end?
6. When you get to the end of this new self imposed plan, how will you know if it's been a good experience?

Keep a copy of your original manuscript notes. I wish I had kept a copy of mine. I can pretty much remember it all though, and have penned this summary for your amusement. Obviously my original document didn't have question 2, but for the sake of completeness I've added a comment to help you.

1.	How did you get here?	Brainstorming my own health dilemma.
2.	How did you end up reading this book about running?	*How did I end up writing this book about running?* I had wanted to read a book like this and I couldn't find one. Recalling the teacher training I did at King's College London, I remembered their motto "in service of society". I decided to write the book!
3.	Why did you get here?	It was at the centre of my Venn diagram, something to match fit, healthy, and cost effective.
4.	What are you hoping to achieve?	Live longer and not kill myself. And stay out of hospital!
5.	Where does it all end?	Not until I die.
6.	When you get to the end of this new self imposed plan, how will you know if it's been a good experience?	My offspring buy into this same philosophy and actively participate in their own health and fitness plan.

Appendix 2 - Example Log

ordinal	date	day	kg	route	km	1/4	1/2	3/4	time	temp	cloud	notes	kmh
735	20241013 0900	Sun	N	Chelmsford Marathon	42.544		156:00		360:14	6>10	80	hills - ran to 10m, yomped to 14m, feeble yomp to 23m, massive effort over last 3 miles with little walking to get a sub 6hr finish - 349m longer than a marathon - effective marathon time 5:57:18	7.086
734	20241009 0715	Wed		London Bridges 10K	10.260	17:05	34:35	52:21	70:21	13		fine - trying for 7min07 - did 6min52 kms	8.751
730	20240928 0730	Sat		Regents Park 400m	2.400				13:08	8	10	started too fast - air cold - heavy breathing - throat sore at end - wanted to eat something - next time bring a banana	10.964
720	20240829 0558	Thu		Vauxhall 15K	15.260	28:52	54:36	82:22	111:26	14>15	40	trying to be a bit slower - achieved that but not by much anyway, slightly slower pace is at least consistent across all quarters	8.217
704	20240808 0628	Thu		London Bridges 10K	10.260	18:20	37:19	56:06	75:33	14>16	2	pace sheet - trying for 7min39 km - did 7min23 km - mouthpiece fell at 10.16k, velcro needs to be fastened fully at start	8.148
700	20240804 0505	Sun	N	London Six Bridges half	21.097	38:18	78:18	116:58	153:15	15>17	99	lots of meh with the new yomping strategy - see diary	8.260
667	20240528 0632	Tue		London Bridges 10K	10.260	15:13	30:02	45:17	60:36	12>13	100	with Koji - he wanted a sub 60min 10k	10.158
662	20240524 0559	Fri		London Bridges 10K	10.260	16:42	32:34	48:55	65:38	10>14	1	knee strain at Oxo tower return - hopped 3 times - stopped - paused for 15/20 secs - resumed slowly	9.379
661	20240519 0605	Sun	N	Fukuoka 15K	16.500	25:17	52:35	81:54	122:00	18>22	1	gentle run with Koji - many stops - photos	8.115
647	20240414 0700	Sun	N	London Bridges 10K	10.260	16:10	32:32	49:08	66:25	9	80	shorts long sleeve top, fewer tourists than 20240331 - that was Easter Sunday!	9.269
638	20240316 1100	Sat		Regents Park 400m	2.400				14:51			TFL meh both ways - should have cycled - run was fine, knee aches a bit this evening 1900 ish - not bad	9.697
611	20231217 0745	Sun	N	London Bridges 10K	10.260	15:58	32:24	49:31	57:01	11	90	too fast - forgot my pace sheet	9.186

Appendix 3 - Example Wiki

A wiki is a type of dynamic and collaborative website whose main feature is that each user can repeatedly edit and manage its content. It's searchable, and it has an inbuilt version control system which allows users to roll back to an older version of the same page. Wikis are popular with teams of people who work remotely. Mine is used within the family, and we have strict access control rules.

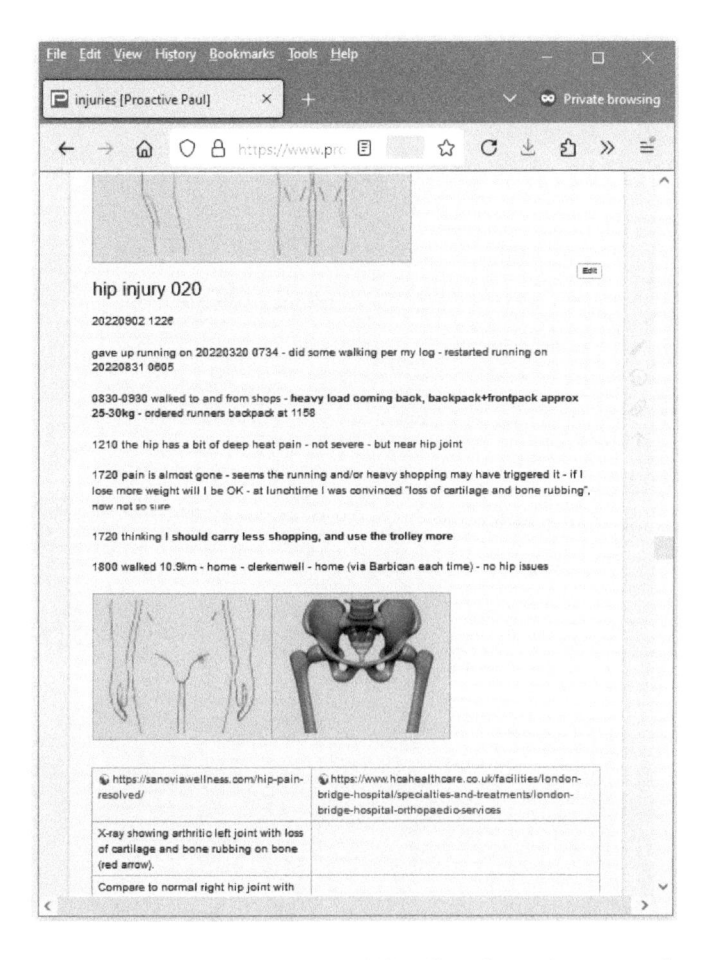

The best known example of a wiki is Wikipedia. If you have a web server you can host your own wiki. Or you can buy into proprietary services. In any case you may want to explore these options (and others):

- Zoho wiki
- DokuWiki
- MediaWiki

Appendix 4 - The Golden Rules

1. Do the warm up routine. — If there's not enough time to do your stretches, then you don't have enough time to do your run. Pulled muscles and torn ligaments are sometimes caused by over exertion of cold, inflexible soft tissue.

2. It's OK to not be OK. — I have done literally hundreds of training runs. My injury log shows that I have abruptly curtailed only a dozen or so. I've walked home slowly a number of times. Only twice in twenty years have I had such a bad injury that I have had to use the bus or the Tube to get home. In central London TFL is a luxury in these circumstances. But as a rule TFL is definitely not a luxury.

3. Cross roads with care. — Do not argue with motor vehicles. They're bigger and stronger than you are, so wait and let them pass, you can get your PB another time. The same thing goes for pedestrian crossings, if in doubt, just stop, and wait for your green light.

4. Avoid manhole covers. — Avoid all manhole covers, and especially avoid the metal ones. My injury log shows several instances where I have awkwardly struck a raised manhole cover or a sunken drain. Just one centimetre above or below the norm is enough to trip me up and that has prematurely ended some of my training runs.

    Ditto, paving stones! If you can see one that's lop sided, avoid it.

5. Avoid wet steps. — I do not run on wet steps, I walk. In fact I walk on all steps at all times even if they're dry. If you've seen the massive staircases at each end of Waterloo Bridge, or Southwark Bridge, then you might recognise the value in slowing down and walking up and down the steps.

6. Your pace is your pace. — I've tried it (and wish I hadn't tried) to keep up with other runners who are faster than me. Occasionally I will slow down and exchange brief words with slower runners, but it's rare that my pace matches others when I'm on a training run. During organised races I sometimes fall into step with others but that only seems to happen after I've covered around two thirds of the distance.

7. Avoid defective surfaces.   If you're a trail runner, you might cope with uneven surfaces, I can't. I like smooth paved surfaces, and I deliberately avoid dodgy, worn out bits of road. If the defective bit is expansive and unavoidable, like the full width of the road (named Upper Ground) between the National Theatre and the Waterloo Imax Cinema then I walk it rather than run it.

8. Run in straight lines.   Be predictable!

When training along the South Bank there are scores of runners. My rule when passing oncoming runners is to adopt a perfectly straight line (usually left of centre, but sometimes right of centre seems more appropriate) and I tend to follow the natural lines of the paving stones. That way the oncoming runner can identify my dominant line and adapt.

We all seem to do it naturally anyway, and it's rare that I need to adjust my line. I've had near misses, but no collisions. In places where there are tight corners (especially on footpaths under bridges) I take the longer outside line, allowing better, faster runners to take the shorter route. I walk the two ridiculously sharp 90° turns at Westminster Bridge by St Thomas' Hospital.

9. Signal.   It happens very little, but sometimes I give a signal like a bike rider does. It helps drivers, pedestrians and other runners understand where I'm going.

By signalling I have definitely avoided one or two collisions with other runners. And I've had one or two bus drivers smile at me too, because all the ambiguity of the encounter has vanished.

Appendix 5 - Example Diary Milton Keynes

Diary entry Sunday 2 Dec 2012

0600 alarm and up
0611 tea + admin
0700 stretches
0715 kit
0721 out
0747 sun up

tracksuit + gloves

Battersea figure of 8

0826 back

miles	1/4	1/2	3/4	time
4.45				55:03

4.79mph - sluggish due to mince pies this week! also been eating more bread less fruit - need to get back to more fruit less bread

park was empty - saw 4 other runners

Appendix 6 - Example Diary Geneva

Diary entry Thursday 14 Dec 2017

0454 up naturally before the alarm
0514 tea, papers, emails

0802 stretches
0811 sun up, minus 2° right now
0816 kit
0828 out

CERN 10k

0940 back

km	1/4	1/2	3/4	time	split 1	split 2
10.27		27:58		**58:05**	27:58	30:07

tracksuit + dayglo + gloves

bright sun, really cold through The Fridge, wanted extra thick gloves, use my regular ones?

frost was lifting at 8k, sunshine makes me happier (and run faster)

only saw 1 other runner, top end of Meyrin

Appendix 7 - Example Diary Chelmsford

Diary entry Tuesday 30 Jul 2024

0500 alarm
0502 up
0510 tea and planning - lots of spreadsheet work

0523 sun up

0536 stretches
0545 kit
0558 out

17 days no run - gentle 7k today - aiming for 6min30 kms

0658 back

km	1/4	1/2	3/4	time	Q1	Q2	Q3	Q4
6.876	12:03	23:37	34:54	**46:37**	12:02	11:34	11:16	11:43

knee dubious for the first 250m - took me 3k to find my stride, then the run was comfortable - 8.85kmh

I overtook 2 runners!! Separate solo runners.

6min47 not 6min30 kms, but that's better than my recent runs, and I had some traffic hold ups on the first quarter

going forward, I will try for 6min30 kms as best I can

Appendix 8 - Example Pace Sheets

kmh >		7.8625	
km	hrs	mins	secs
1		7	39
2		15	17
3		22	56
4		30	34
5		38	12
6		45	51
7		53	29
8	1	1	8
9	1	8	46
10	1	16	24
11	1	24	3
12	1	31	41
13	1	39	20
14	1	46	58
15	1	54	36
16	2	2	15
17	2	9	53
18	2	17	32
19	2	25	10
20	2	32	48
21	2	40	27
22	2	48	5
23	2	55	44
24	3	3	22
25	3	11	0
26	3	18	39
27	3	26	17
28	3	33	56
29	3	41	34
30	3	49	12
31	3	56	51
32	4	4	29
33	4	12	8
34	4	19	46
35	4	27	24
36	4	35	3
37	4	42	41
38	4	50	20
39	4	57	58
40	5	5	36
41	5	13	15
42	5	20	53
42.2	5	22	23

mph >		4.88	
mile	hrs	mins	secs
1		12	18
2		24	35
3		36	53
4		49	10
5	1	1	27
6	1	13	45
7	1	26	2
8	1	38	20
9	1	50	37
10	2	2	54
11	2	15	12
12	2	27	29
13	2	39	47
14	2	52	4
15	3	4	21
16	3	16	39
17	3	28	56
18	3	41	14
19	3	53	31
20	4	5	48
21	4	18	6
22	4	30	23
23	4	42	41
24	4	54	58
25	5	7	15
26	5	19	33
26.22	5	22	14

Appendix 9 - Race Day Checklist

Items under advance prep (like safety pins for attaching your bib) may need to be bought ahead of time. They're on the checklist in order to avoid a last minute panic!

Two meals are carried, in case a simple second breakfast is needed if you arrive at the venue long before the race starts. Afterwards, a home made packed lunch may prove more satisfying than any fast food in the event village.

Lots of small plastic bags are useful after the race, for wet clothes or dirty shoes and the like. Sturdy elastic bands will keep them closed so that they don't interfere with other stuff.

Advance prep

- lipsalve
- sun cream
- moisturiser
- energy gel
- chocolate
- train tickets
- pace sheet
- safety pins
- charge phone

Backpack

- cash
- credit card
- sun cream
- lipsalve
- tracksuit trousers
- train tickets
- travel card
- baseball cap
- energy gel x20
- clean filled bladder
- phone
- keys

Kit

shoes	gloves
socks	sweat band
shorts	mini towel
T shirt	watch
long sleeved top	pace sheet
dayglo jacket	bib + chip

Drop bag

trainers	gloves
socks	soap
pants	towel
trousers	plastic bags
shirt	elastic bands
long sleeved top	power bank
jacket	charging cable

Breakfast and lunch

apple	apple
clementine	clementine
banana	banana
	sandwich
	chocolate bar
	flask of tea

Bibliography

Atkinson, J. (1966) *A Theory of Achievement Motivation* New York: Robert E Krieger Publishing

Augar, P. et al, (2019). *Review of Post-18 Education and Funding: Independent Panel Report.* London: Her Majesty's Stationery Office

Backley, S. (2006) *The Champion in All of Us*. Brands Hatch, UK: May 2006 [Unpublished item]

Bloom, S. et al, (2007) Effects of exercise on gut peptides, energy intake and appetite. *Journal of Endocrinology*, (193/2) pp251-258

Bogl, L.H. et al, (2009) Improving the Accuracy of Self-Reports on Diet and Physical Exercise: The Co-Twin Control Method. *Twin Research and Human Genetics* 12(6), pp.531–540. Available at: http://www.ncbi.nlm.nih.gov/pubmed/19943715 (Accessed 5 Apr 2023)

Booth, F.W. et al, (2012). Lack of exercise is a major cause of chronic diseases. *Comprehensive Physiology*, 2(2), pp1143-1211.

Bregman, P. (2018) "How to Actually Start the Task You've Been Avoiding" *Harvard Business Review* 30 May 2018 (2018/5) pp t84-t86

Bruch, H. (1957) *The Importance of Overweight* New York: WW Norton & Company

Bruch, H. (1973) *Eating Disorders: Obesity, Anorexia Nervosa, and the Person within*: New York: Basic Books

Canguilhem, G. (1966) *Le Normal et le Pathologique.* Paris: Presses Universitaires de France

Canguilhem, G. (1989) *The Normal and the Pathological.* Translated from the French by C. Fawcett. Brooklyn, USA: Zone Books

Checkland, P. (1999) *Systems Thinking, Systems Practice* Hoboken, New Jersey, USA: Wiley

Covey, S. (2020) *The 7 Habits Of Highly Effective People* London: Simon & Schuster

Das, S. & Ungoed-Thomas, J. (2023) *"Skinny jab drug firm facing fresh inquiries after serious breaches of industry code"* Available at: https://www.theguardian.com/business/2023/mar/18/skinny-jab-drug-firm-facing-fresh-inquiries-after-breach-of-industry-code (Accessed 8 April 2023)

Davies, C. (2011) *World's oldest marathon runner completes Toronto race at age 100.* Available at https://www.theguardian.com/uk/2011/oct/17/worlds-oldest-marathon-runner-100 (Accessed: 24 Dec 2017)

Descartes, R. (1912) *Discourse on Method.* Translated from the Latin by I. Maclean. London: J M Dent & Sons

Deitrick, B. (1999) *"WMA Road age-grading calculator"* Available at: http://www.howardgrubb.co.uk/athletics/wmaroad15.html (Accessed 7 Feb 2023)

Drucker, P. (1974) *Management: Tasks, Responsibilities, Practices.* New York: Butterworth Heinemann

Duffy, J. (2018) *Strava Review* Available at: https://www.pcmag.com/reviews/strava (Accessed 8 Feb 2023)

Edwards, S. & Gately, P. *Outcomes at 1 year in a community tier 3 weight management service* Obesity Reviews 23,52 on 25 Oct 2002 available at https://onlinelibrary.wiley.com/toc/1467789x/2022/23/S2 (accessed 2 Apr 2023)

The Economist (2015) *Style Guide 2015* Available at: https://cdn.static-economist.com/sites/default/files/store/Style_Guide_2015.pdf (Accessed: 27 April 2020)

The Economist (2023) *New drugs could spell an end to the world's obesity epidemic* Available at: https://www.economist.com/leaders/2023/03/02/new-drugs-could-spell-an-end-to-the-worlds-obesity-epidemic (Accessed: 11 March 2023)

Ellson, A. (2022) *More than 42m UK adults will be overweight by 2040.* Available at: https://www.theguardian.com/society/2022/may/19/more-than-42m-uk-adults-will-be-overweight-by-2040 (Accessed: 3 November 2022)

Fennell, R. (ed) *Problem solving.* Hull, UK: DDD North, 3 Dec 2022 [Unpublished item]

Ford, P. (ed.) *The unofficial story of medical practice in England 1500–1800.* London: Royal College of Physicians, 3 Oct 2024 [Unpublished item]

Franklin, B. (1793) *The Autobiography of Benjamin Franklin* London: J Parsons

Galbraith-Emami, S. & Lobstein, T (2013) The impact of initiatives to limit the advertising of food and beverage products to children. *Obesity Reviews*, 14 (2) pp960-974

Goater, J. & Melvin, D. (2012) *The Art of Running Faster, Improve technique, training and performance.* Champaign, USA: Human Kinetics

Greger, M. (2017) *How Not To Die.* London: Macmillan

Gregory, A. (2022) *YouGov health survey portrays nation of tired, overweight layabouts.* Available at: https://www.thetimes.co.uk/article/yougov-health-survey-portrays-nation-of-tired-overweight-layabouts-g8dm97w08 (Accessed: 3 November 2022)

Griffiths, A.(2020) *A Geeks Guide to People.* Available at: https://www.youtube.com/watch?v=jCStTpKWBMc (Accessed: 12 December 2020)

Haskell, W.L. et al (2007). Physical activity and public health: Updated recommendation for adults from the American College of Sports Medicine and the American Heart Association. *Medicine and Science in Sports and Exercise*, 39(8), pp1423-1434

Higdon, H. (2020) *Marathon: The Ultimate Training Guide: Advice, Plans, and Programs for Half and Full Marathons.* New York: Harmony/Rodale

Hilton, P. (2022) *How to stay fit over 50? Stop training like a 20-year-old* Available at: https://www.thetimes.co.uk/article/how-to-stay-fit-over-50-tips-for-training-hx0rsz6rn (Accessed: 13 August 2022)

Howard, C. (2012) *Special report: Obesity* Available at: http://www.economist.com/news/special-report/21568065-world-getting-wider-says-charlotte-howard-what-can-be-done-about-it-big (Accessed: 15 December 2012)

Jewell, T. (2020) *The Best Healthy Lifestyle Apps of 2020* Available at: https://www.healthline.com/health/mental-health/top-healthy-lifestyle-iphone-android-apps (Accessed 7 Feb 2023)

Jurek, S. (2012) *Eat & Run, An Unlikely Journey to Ultramarathon Greatness.* London: Bloomsbury

Kaplan, R. and Norton, D. (1992). The Balanced Scorecard – Measures That Drive Performance. *Harvard Business Review* (January–February) pp71-79.

Kawahara, D. (2022) *Habits Influence Our Behavior More Than We Realize* Available at: https://www.verywellmind.com/study-finds-we-underestimate-influence-of-habits-when-explaining-our-behavior-5271093 (Accessed 4 Oct 2024)

Kuhn, T. (1962) *The Structure of Scientific Revolutions* Chicago: University of Chicago Press

Lally, P. (2010) "How are habits formed: Modelling habit formation in the real world". *European Journal of Social Psychology* (40/6) pp998-1009

The Lancet (2009) What is health? The ability to adapt. *The Lancet,* 373(9666), p781.

Laursen, B. and Veenstra, R. (2021) Toward understanding the functions of peer influence. *The Journal of Research on Adolescence* (31/4) pp889-907.

Macrotrends (2023) *U.K. Population 1950-2023* Available at: https://www.macrotrends.net/countries/GBR/united-kingdom/population (Accessed: 16 April 2023)

Maltz, M. (1960) *Psycho-Cybernetics: A New Way to Get More Living out of Life,* New York: Prentice-Hall

Maxted, C. (2024) *The Ultimate Ultra Running Handbook.* London: Bloomsbury

McGuire, J. (2019) *What is the average marathon finish time?* Available at: https://www.runnersworld.com/uk/training/marathon/a27787958/average-marathon-finish-time/ (Accessed: 3 Oct 2024)

McPartland, D. et al (2010). *Nelson Physical Education Studies For WA.* Melbourne, Australia: Cengage Learning.

National Health Service (2023) *"Keeping active guidelines"* Available at: https://www.nhsinform.scot/healthy-living/keeping-active/keeping-active-guidelines (Accessed 6 April 2023)

Nolsoe, E. (2021) *Half of English people say they're overweight, obese or morbidly obese; the NHS says it's two thirds.* Available at: https://yougov.co.uk/topics/health/articles-reports/2021/07/20/half-english-people-say-theyre-overweight-obese-or (Accessed: 3 November 2022)

Olima, P. (2021) *Fit, Smash Your Goals and Stay Strong for Life.* London: Simon & Schuster

Orbach, S. (2023) *Weight Watchers wins when our diets fail* Available at: https://www.theguardian.com/commentisfree/2023/mar/16/weight-watchers-diet-society-food-industry-customer (Accessed: 9 April 2023)

Orwell, G. (1946) *Politics and the English Language.* London: Renard Press

Our Future Health (2021) *Our Future Health Governance Manual* Available at: https://ourfuturehealth.org.uk/wp-content/uploads/2022/01/Our-Future-Health-governance-manual-December-2021.pdf (Accessed: 24 October 2022)

Oxley, J. (2022) *The crisis at the heart of the Conservative party* Available at: https://www.spectator.co.uk/article/the-crisis-at-the-heart-of-the-modern-conservative-party (Accessed: 11 Aug 2022)

Petley, S. (2007) *New money is last hope in battle to save rainforests* Available at: https://www.theguardian.com/business/2007/oct/14/money.environment (Accessed: 20 Mar 2019)

Plato et al. (2021) *Republic.* Translated from the Greek by D. Lee. London: Harper Collins

Piaget, J. (1982) *Consensus and Controversy.* Lavenham, UK: The Lavenham Press

Rosling, H. et al (2019) *Factfulness: Ten Reasons We're Wrong About The World.* London: Sceptre

Shepherd, J. (2006) *The Complete Guide to Sports Training.* London: A&C Black Publishers

Skinner, B. (1953) *Science and Human Behavior.* New York: Simon & Schuster

Spiegelman, B. and Flier, J (2001) "Obesity and the regulation of energy balance". *Cell* 23 Feb 2001 (104/4) pp531-43

Taubes, G. (2021) *How a 'fatally, tragically flawed' paradigm has derailed the science of obesity* Available at: https://www.statnews.com/2021/09/13/how-a-fatally-tragically-flawed-paradigm-has-derailed-the-science-of-obesity/ (Accessed: 28 February 2023)

Tedstone, A. (2018) *Putting healthier food environments at the heart of planning.* Available at https://ukhsa.blog.gov.uk/2018/06/29/putting-healthier-food-environments-at-the-heart-of-planning/ (Accessed: 8 Dec 2021)

The Times Editorial (2022) *The Times view on Our Future Health programme: Speak Your Weight* Available at: https://www.thetimes.co.uk/article/the-times-view-on-our-future-health-programme-speak-your-weight-lzk0lmxjp (Accessed: 24 October 2022)

Trembath, R. (ed.) *King's Health Partners.* London: King's College London Impact Reception, 14 Jun 2023 [Unpublished item]

van Tulleken, C. (2023) *Ultra-Processed People: Why Do We All Eat Stuff That Isn't Food.* London: Cornerstone Press

Vassos, A. (2021) *How to Run a Marathon. The Go-to Guide for Anyone and Everyone.* London: Harper-Collins

Warburton, D.E. et al (2006) Health benefits of physical activity: The evidence. *Canadian Medical Association Journal*, 174(6), pp801-809.

Wharton-Malcolm, C. (2024) *All You Need is Rhythm & Grit.* London: Souvenir Press

World Health Organisation (2021) *Obesity and overweight* Available at: https://www.who.int/news-room/fact-sheets/detail/obesity-and-overweight (Accessed 1 April 2023)

World Health Organisation (2022) *Physical activity* Available at: https://www.who.int/news-room/fact-sheets/detail/physical-activity (Accessed 6 April 2023)

World Health Organisation (2023) *Obesity* Available at: https://www.who.int/health-topics/obesity#tab=tab_1 (Accessed 1 April 2023)

World Masters Athletics (2016) *WMA Road age-grading calculator* Available at: http://www.howardgrubb.co.uk/athletics/wmaroad15.html (Accessed 7 Feb 2023)

Yeo, G. (2021) *BMI: We know it's flawed* Available at: https://www.sciencefocus.com/comment/bmi-we-know-its-flawed-so-why-do-we-still-use-it/ (Accessed 19 June 2021)

Yeo, G. (2021) *Why Calories Don't Count: How we got the science of weight loss wrong.* London: Orion Spring

Zulqarnain, A. (2016) *How To Run A Marathon: Absolutely for beginners who never run a marathon before.* Available at: https://www.amazon.co.uk/How-Run-Marathon-Absolutely-beginners-ebook/dp/B01N0EAYMW/ (Downloaded: 22 Feb 2024)

Index

100 year old, 182
400m track, 44-45, 141, 182

AeT, 144
alcohol, 139-140
artist (inspirational), 3-4

Backley J, 1, 67, 74, 178
Backley S, 1-2, 5
backpack, 17-19, 81-83, 90-94, 107-109, 157-158
Bexley Heath, 1-2
Birmingham, 106-107
blister, 23-24
blood pressure, 5, 133-134, 183
BMA, 133
BMI, 35, 79, 87, 111, 127-128, 133, 143
BMJ, 21, 134
Boston, 112-113, 119, 121, 159, 178
Brighton, 55-57, 61-62, 65

calories, 76, 125-134, 139-140, 144, 160
Canguilhem G, 41, 53, 119, 134, 146, 185
carb loading, 58, 121, 142-143, 159-160, 165, 169
Chelmsford, x, 28, 118-122, 141, 180-181, 163-164, 169-179, 184
Close C, 3-4
clothing, 10-11, 16-17, 19, 29, 59-60, 105, 134, 164, 169
   pants, 14
   shirts, 15
   shorts, 15
   socks, 14
   wet weather, 19, 118, 167
coach, ix, 2, 12, 33-387, 39, 137, 160, 182
Confucius, 6, 129, 140
Covey S, 55

Daleks, 73
Descartes R, xii, 41
DEXA, 127
diet, 6, 53, 116, 126-131, 145, 159
    fads, 127, 130, 134
    Japan, 132, 169
    slimming aids, 134
    suspension of, 143
dopamine, 9, 120, 138
Drucker P, 34, 183
ducks, 176

energy gel, 68-69, 76, 110, 144, 155-158, 171-172

fartlek, 137, 145
fat max, 144
fictitious characters, 84-85, 151
fish & chips, 125
Franklin B, 4

Geneva, x, 17, 24-26, 38, 44, 79-86, 89-103, 105-106, 130, 184
gluconeogenesis, 142
glycogen, 121, 142-145, 155-156, 164
goal setting, ix, 3, 39, 55-57, 150, 183
Gravesend, 66
Great North Run, 109-110
gym, ix-x, 1-5, 12-13, 26-37, 56

habits, 10, 21, 29, 39, 55, 113, 126, 140, 153-154
humour, 84-85, 151-152, 176

IAAF, 171, 178
injury, ix, 5, 11, 21, 178
    log, 140, 183
    lower limb, 107-120
    prevention, 28-29, 41, 153
    RSI, 53

   stress fracture, 114-116
interval training, 137, 144-145, 159, 164, 189

Japan, xi
   diet, 132, 169
   Rajio Taiso, 181
   routes, 5, 80, 119
   runner, 99
   shopping, 17, 23-24, 28

Kawahara D, 153
King's College London, 125, 137-138, 146

life long learning, 137-138, 144-146
Loch Ness, 118-121
log, 2-6, 10, 36-39, 55, 108, 150, 183
   blood pressure, 134
   distance, 13, 36, 58, 61
   habits, 38-39
   shoes (adverse), 23-26
   stretches & exercises, 51, 79
   weight loss, 35, 125-126, 140
London Marathon, 55, 65, 75, 184-186

metabolism, 144, 155, 178
Milton Keynes, x, 61-62, 65-76, 79-80, 86, 96-98, 105-108, 141-143, 155, 183

Naismith W, 172-173

obesity, 9, 35, 53, 79, 133
Olima P, 137
Olympic Games, 2, 50, 55, 75, 113
Oxley J, 39

pace, 28, 36-39, 56, 61, 71-74, 83-84, 112-116, 119-120, 145, 151, 158, 185
   golden rule, 199
   pace setters, 83-84, 89-92, 97, 163, 169-171, 175, 178

pace sheet, 84, 112, 163, 166-167, 169, 209
   rehearse, 114, 158
Peterborough, 112-113, 119
Plato, 138

Raube K, 128
Royal Air Force, 43-45, 190
Royal Institution, 127
Royal Marines, 45-46
RSI, 53
Runners World, 33-34, 36, 62, 145

Salford University, 138
Shepherd J, 137
shoes, 10-14, 21-30
   Adidas, 12-13, 21
   Brooks, 27
   fold test, 29-30
   New Balance, 13-14, 22-25
   Nike, 25-28
   Reebok, 12-13, 21
Stormtroopers, 67-69
stretches, 28, 39, 41-53, 170, 181, 199
swimming, 2-3, 36, 44, 100, 113, 184

tapering, 160-161
Tonbridge, 111-112, 120, 175, 178
Toronto, 182
Tracey B, 33
treadmill
   gym, 2-5, 12-13, 36
   shoe shopping, 24-25
Trembath R, 125, 127, 134, 146
Triffids, 72-73, 185
van Tulleken C, 128-132

ultra processed food, 128-129, 132, 185
University College London, 153

velo park, 66
Venn diagram, 9
visioning, 2, 160-161, 177

wall (hitting the), 121, 141-143, 149, 173
weight management *see* "calories"
Wharton-Malcolm C, 137
wiki, 4-5, 145-146, 183, 197
Wokingham, 59-60, 69, 118

Yeo G, 42, 127-129, 134, 144-146, 155, 189
yomp
   Chelmsford, 169, 173-175
   Geneva, 97-101
   Milton Keynes, 70-73
   origins, 45-46
   strategy, 119-120, 141, 164

BV - #0027 - 061124 - C0 - 229/152/14 - PB - 9781068550904 - Matt Lamination